ENTREPRENEURSHIP IN AYURVEDA

Exploring Vast Business Opportunities in Ancient Healing Science

Dr. Mukesh Aggarwal

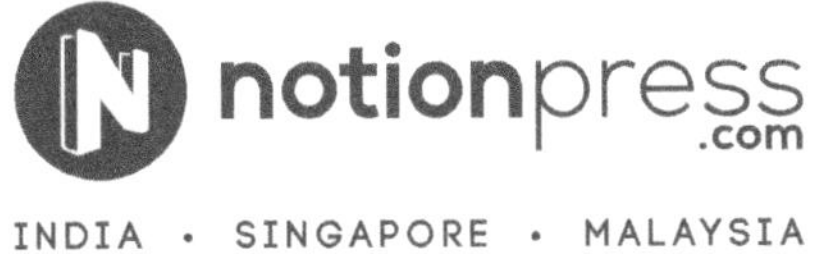

INDIA · SINGAPORE · MALAYSIA

ISBN 979-8-89186-778-9

Foreword

PROF. VAIDYA KARTAR SINGH DHIMAN
VICE CHANCELLOR
Ph.D., M.D. (Ay.), CHM, FRAV
प्रो. वैद्य करतार सिंह धीमान
कुलपति

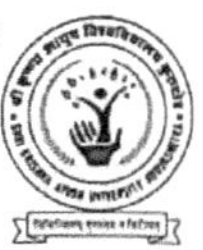

SHRI KRISHNA AYUSH UNIVERSITY,
KURUKSHETRA - 136118 (INDIA)
(Established by the Haryana State Legislature Act-25 of 2017)
श्री कृष्णा आयुष विश्वविद्यालय,
कुरुक्षेत्र - 136118 हरियाणा (भारत)
(हरियाणा राज्य विधान सभा अधिनियम संख्या 25/2017 द्वारा स्थापित)

No.SKAU/VC/2023/1051
Dated: 07.11.2023

FOREWARD

I am delighted to pen the foreword for "Entrepreneurship in Ayurveda: Exploring Vast Business Opportunities in Ancient Healing Science" by Dr. Mukesh Aggarwal. This book is a commendable effort that not only aligns with the resurgence of Ayurveda but also encapsulates the essence of Ayurvedic entrepreneurship in a manner that is both enlightening and insightful.

Ayurveda, the science of life, has been a cornerstone of holistic health for millennia. In a world where the pursuit of well-being has become paramount, the principles of Ayurveda offer an extraordinary pathway to achieving physical, mental, and spiritual balance. Dr. Aggarwal's book is a timely and invaluable resource for those who seek to harness the potential of Ayurveda in the realm of entrepreneurship.

This book is divided into three sections, each focusing on a vital aspect of Ayurvedic entrepreneurship. From laying the foundation and understanding the core principles of Ayurveda to delving into market analysis and identifying business opportunities, it comprehensively covers the landscape. Chapters like Ayurveda Hospitals and Clinics, Manufacturing Units, Tourism and Hospitality, Trading, Herbs Agriculture, Research, Education, and Publishing provide a holistic view of the diverse avenues within Ayurveda entrepreneurship.

Furthermore, Dr. Aggarwal offers guidance on building and scaling an Ayurveda venture, addressing regulatory frameworks, advocating eco-friendliness, and discussing the future of Ayurveda. The inclusion of case studies of successful Ayurveda ventures and a rich resource index adds practical value to the book, making it an indispensable reference for budding entrepreneurs and seasoned practitioners alike.

As the Vice-Chancellor of Kurukshetra Ayurveda University, I have witnessed the remarkable resurgence of Ayurveda both nationally and globally. It is heartening to see a book that not only celebrates this resurgence but also acts as a guiding light for those who wish to embrace Ayurveda as a vocation. Ayurveda is not just a science; but a art of life. It,not only promotes wellness, health and healing but also offers immense opportunities for innovation, growth, and entrepreneurship.

Dr. Mukesh Aggarwal's expertise and dedication to Ayurveda shine through the pages of this book. His extensive knowledge and passion for this ancient healing science are evident in every word. I wholeheartedly endorse this book and believe that it will inspire and empower individuals to embark on a transformative journey into the world of Ayurvedic entrepreneurship.

I hope that readers find this book as enlightening and inspiring as I have, and I encourage you to explore the vast business opportunities that Ayurveda has to offer. May this book serve as a catalyst for the resurgence of Ayurveda in the entrepreneurial landscape, benefiting not only the individuals who embark on this journey but also the countless individuals who will benefit from the healing touch of Ayurveda.

7.11.2023
Prof. Vaidya Kartar Singh Dhiman

Preface

"Ayurveda teaches us to live in harmony with ourselves, others, and the environment to achieve true well-being."

Acharya Charak

Ayurveda, the ancient science of healing, has experienced a renaissance in recent years. It is not merely a system of traditional medicine but a profound philosophy that encompasses the holistic well-being of the individual. This resurgence is not limited to the realms of health and wellness; it extends to the world of entrepreneurship.

The pages that follow are a comprehensive guide to understanding the potential, opportunities, and challenges that exist within the vast landscape of Ayurveda entrepreneurship. The journey we are about to embark on is one that combines the wisdom of the ages with the innovative spirit of modern business.

In today's world, where the pursuit of health, balance, and sustainability is a common aspiration, Ayurveda is a guiding light. It offers a path to not only a prosperous business but also a meaningful one. This book takes you on a journey through the rich history, principles, and contemporary relevance of Ayurveda, while also providing practical insights into various avenues where Ayurveda can be integrated into entrepreneurship.

From establishing Ayurveda healthcare centers to cultivating organic herbs, and from blending Ayurveda with tourism to venturing into the digital realm, there are numerous opportunities waiting to be explored. You will also discover the importance of regulatory frameworks, sustainable practices, and the role of technology in shaping the future of Ayurveda entrepreneurship.

Throughout this book, I have strived to offer you a holistic perspective on the subject. It's not just about making profits; it's about making a positive impact on people's lives. "Ayurveda Ventures" should resonate with your passion for health, well-being, and the timeless wisdom of this ancient science.

I hope this book serves as a guiding light for those who wish to venture into the fascinating world of Ayurveda entrepreneurship. May it inspire you to embark on a journey filled with promise and potential, and may it contribute to the continued growth and recognition of Ayurveda on a global scale.

Dr. Mukesh Aggarwal

www.mukeshaggarwal.com

Acknowledgments

I extend my heartfelt gratitude to the individuals and institutions who have played an invaluable role in the creation of this book. Without their support, guidance, and contributions, this project would not have been possible.

I would like to express my deepest appreciation to:

Prof (Vaidya) K.S. Dhiman: For providing the forward and sharing his wisdom and expertise as the Vice Chancellor of Ayurveda University, Kurukshetra and formed Director General of Central Council for Research in Ayurvedic Sciences (CCRAS)

My Family: For their unwavering support and encouragement throughout this journey.

Contributors and Experts: To the numerous Ayurveda experts, practitioners, and entrepreneurs who generously shared their insights and experiences.

Readers and Ayurveda Enthusiasts: For their enthusiasm and interest in promoting Ayurveda entrepreneurship.

Research Partners: Those who assisted in data collection, analysis, and case studies.

Publishers and Editors: For their dedication and expertise in bringing this book to fruition.

Well-wishers: Everyone who believed in the importance of Ayurveda entrepreneurship and its potential for holistic wellness.

I am grateful to each one of you for being a part of this endeavor.

With gratitude,

Dr. Mukesh Aggarwal

Contents

Section III
Building and Scaling Your Ayurveda Venture

Case Studies of
Various Successful Ayurveda Ventures

Section-1

Foundation of Ayurveda Entrepreneurship

Chapter 1

Introduction

प्रयोजनं चास्य स्वस्थस्य स्वास्थ्यरक्षणमातुरस्य विकार
प्रशमनंच॥२६॥

Prayojanaṃ cāsya svasthasya svāsthyarakṣaṇamāturasya vikārapraśamanaṃ

The utility of Ayurveda is to maintain the health of a healthy individual and heal the disease of the sick.

Charaka Sutrasthana, Chapter 30, verse 26

HIGHLIGHTS

Ayurveda's resurgence is fueled by holistic health, sustainability, mainstream integration, global accessibility, and scientific validation.

The book outlines its purpose to explore Ayurveda's resurgence and provides a broad scope covering topics like history, market analysis, healthcare facilities, manufacturing, tourism, trading, herbs farming, research, education, publishing, regulatory aspects, business models, and ethical practices.

RESURGENCE OF AYURVEDA

Ayurveda, the ancient system of natural medicine that originated in India over 5,000 years ago, is experiencing a remarkable resurgence in the modern world. This resurgence can be attributed to a variety of factors, including a growing interest in holistic health, the desire for natural and sustainable healthcare solutions, and the integration of Ayurvedic principles into mainstream medicine. Here, we will explore the reasons behind the resurgence of Ayurveda and its potential to bridge the gap between ancient wisdom and modern healthcare.

Holistic Health and Wellness

One of the key drivers behind the resurgence of Ayurveda is the growing emphasis on holistic health and wellness. Ayurveda, which focuses on the balance of mind, body, and spirit, aligns well with this trend. Modern individuals are increasingly seeking comprehensive approaches to health that go beyond symptom management and address the root causes of health issues. Ayurveda's personalized treatment plans, which consider an individual's unique constitution and lifestyle make it an attractive option for those seeking holistic well-being.

Natural and Sustainable Healthcare

Ayurveda's emphasis on natural remedies and sustainable healthcare practices is another factor contributing to its resurgence. In a world where synthetic drugs and invasive treatments are common, Ayurveda offers a more gentle and eco-friendly approach. Ayurvedic therapies often involve the use of herbs, diet, and lifestyle modifications, minimizing the environmental impact and reducing the risk of side effects associated with pharmaceuticals.

Integration into Mainstream Medicine

Ayurveda is no longer confined to the fringes of alternative medicine. It is increasingly being integrated into mainstream healthcare systems. In India, for example, there are Ayurvedic hospitals and institutions that work alongside allopathic (Western) medicine to offer a holistic approach to patient care. This integration recognizes the potential of Ayurveda in complementing modern medical practices and expanding treatment options.

Globalization and Information Accessibility

The globalization of knowledge through the internet and the ease of information accessibility have played a significant role in Ayurveda's resurgence. Individuals worldwide can now learn about Ayurveda, access Ayurvedic practitioners, and even order Ayurvedic products online. The democratization of information has empowered people to explore and adopt traditional healing systems like Ayurveda.

Scientific Validation and Research

Modern scientific research is beginning to validate many Ayurvedic principles and practices. Studies are confirming the efficacy of Ayurvedic herbs, treatments, and dietary guidelines. This scientific validation adds credibility to Ayurveda and helps bridge the gap between ancient wisdom and modern healthcare.

Conclusion

The resurgence of Ayurveda represents a convergence of ancient wisdom and modern healthcare needs. With its focus on holistic well-being, natural and sustainable healthcare, integration into mainstream medicine and the support of scientific research, Ayurveda is well-positioned to play a more prominent role in the healthcare landscape of the 21st century. This resurgence reflects a growing recognition that traditional systems of medicine, like Ayurveda, can complement and enhance modern healthcare, providing individuals with more choices and personalized approaches to their well-being. As the world continues to seek a balance between ancient wisdom and modern advancements, Ayurveda's resurgence is set to flourish.

PURPOSE AND SCOPE OF THE BOOK

The purpose and scope of the book "ENTREPRENEURSHIP IN AYURVEDA: Exploring Vast Business Opportunities in Ancient Healing" are multifaceted, aiming to provide an extensive guide for individuals and entrepreneurs interested in the world of Ayurveda and its vast business opportunities.

The primary purpose of this book is to shed light on the resurgence of Ayurveda in the contemporary world. Ayurveda, an ancient system of holistic healing that originated in India, has been gaining increasing global recognition and popularity. This resurgence is driven by the growing demand for natural and holistic health solutions in a world where conventional medicine often falls short. The book seeks to explore the reasons behind this resurgence, highlighting the increasing interest in traditional and holistic healing practices.

The scope of the book is broad, encompassing various aspects of Ayurveda entrepreneurship, with a comprehensive structure consisting of seventeen sections. These sections cover a wide array of topics, ranging from understanding the historical roots and philosophy of Ayurveda to delving into Ayurvedic market analysis. The book explores the current local and global trends in Ayurveda and identifies niche areas and market gaps, providing invaluable insights for those seeking to establish businesses in this field.

Additionally, the book offers detailed guidance on setting up Ayurveda healthcare facilities, including state-of-the-art hospitals, specialized clinics, beauty clinics, and wellness centers. It delves into Ayurvedic manufacturing units, explaining the processes behind classical and proprietary formulations, skin and beauty care products, dietary supplements, herbal extracts, and even Ayurvedic veterinary medicines.

Ayurveda's potential in the tourism and hospitality industry is also thoroughly explored, as the book discusses the establishment of wellness resorts and the fusion of tourism with traditional Ayurvedic treatments. Moreover, it delves into trading in Ayurveda through physical retail stores and online e-commerce platforms, as well as the export of Ayurvedic herbs and medicines.

The book emphasizes the importance of Ayurvedic herbs farming, focusing on cultivating and selling organic herbs and plants, thus promoting sustainable practices and supporting local communities.

Furthermore, it addresses Ayurveda research and innovation, encouraging entrepreneurs to develop new products and treatment methodologies, along with innovative equipment and software for diagnosis and treatment. It highlights the need for educational and training institutes in the field, explaining the process of establishing Ayurvedic colleges and training institutes and designing online certificate courses for practitioners and the general public.

The book also delves into the world of publishing and digital media, guiding readers on creating Ayurveda content through books, e-books, magazines, YouTube, blogs, and mobile apps for online consultation. It discusses the regulatory framework surrounding Ayurveda in India and globally, ensuring that readers are aware of the legal and quality control aspects of this industry.

In the final sections, the book provides entrepreneurial insights, including various business models and case studies of successful Ayurveda ventures. It details the steps to launch an Ayurveda venture, strategies for funding and investment, as well as marketing and branding techniques for building a trusted brand in the Ayurveda space. The book also underscores the importance of ethical and sustainable practices in Ayurveda businesses and reflects on the future of Ayurveda, including emerging trends and the role of technology.

In conclusion, "ENTREPRENEURSHIP IN AYURVEDA: Exploring Vast Business Opportunities in Ancient Healing" serves as a comprehensive guide, equipping readers with the knowledge, insights, and strategies to enter the world of Ayurveda entrepreneurship successfully. Its purpose is to empower individuals to harness the potential of Ayurveda in the modern business landscape, and its scope is extensive, covering all aspects of this holistic and thriving industry.

*****

Chapter 2

Understanding Ayurveda

हिताहितं सुखं दुःखमायुस्तस्य हिताहितम्|
मानं च तच्च यत्रोक्तमायुर्वेदः स उच्यते||४१||

Hitahitam sukham dukhamayustasya hitahitam
Maanam cha tacha yatrokatmayurvedah sa uchyate

Ayurveda is the science of life. Ayurveda gives remedies for…

Hitayu – an advantageous life

Ahita Ayu – a disadvantageous life

Sukhayu – a happy state of health and mind

Ahitayu – an unhappy state of health and mind.

It also explains what is good and bad for life and how to measure life.

Charaka Sutra Sthana, Chapter 1, verse 41

HIGHLIGHTS

Ayurveda is based on three bio energies, holistic well-being, and a focus on prevention and balance.

Ayurveda principles Tridosha Theory, Panchamahabhutas, Prakriti, Vikriti, Sapta-Dhatus, Agni, Malas, Srotas, Ama, Rasayana and Vajikarana therapies, lifestyle and diet, herbal medicine, yoga and meditation, all aimed at individualized well-being.

HISTORICAL ROOTS OF AYURVEDA

Ayurveda, often referred to as the "Science of Life," has deep historical roots that date back thousands of years. Its origins can be traced to the Indian subcontinent, and its development is intertwined with the cultural, philosophical, and medical history of the region.

The foundations of Ayurveda can be found in ancient Indian texts known as the Vedas, particularly the Rigveda and Atharvaveda, which are among the oldest known scriptures in the world, dating back to around 1500 BCE. These texts contain references to various herbs and healing practices, laying the groundwork for Ayurveda.

The earliest comprehensive text dedicated to Ayurvedic principles and practices is the "Charaka Samhita," attributed to the sage Charaka. This text, believed to have been composed between the 6th and 2nd centuries BCE, provides a systematic framework for understanding health, disease, and the use of natural remedies. It categorizes diseases, classifies herbs and minerals, and outlines principles of diagnosis and treatment.

Another foundational text is the "Sushruta Samhita," attributed to Sushruta, who is regarded as the father of surgery in Ayurveda. This text, dated to a similar period as the Charaka Samhita, details surgical techniques and medical procedures, including plastic surgery and the use of surgical instruments.

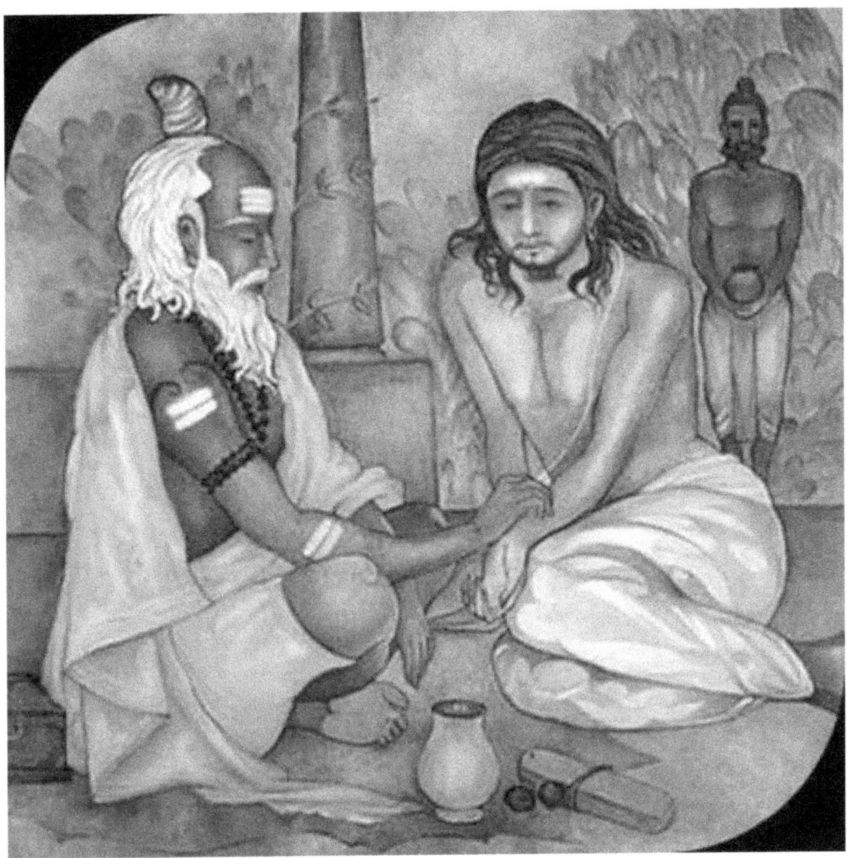

Fig: 2.1 Ancient Ayurvedacharya treating patient

Over time, Ayurveda continued to evolve, absorbing influences from other cultures, including Greek and Persian medicine. It flourished during the Gupta period (around 4th to 6th centuries CE) and continued to be influential throughout India's history.

During the medieval and colonial periods, Ayurveda faced challenges, but it has experienced resurgence in the modern era, both in India and globally. It's been integrated with contemporary medicine, and its holistic approach to health and well-being has gained recognition and popularity.

In conclusion, the historical roots of Ayurveda are deeply embedded in the ancient traditions of the Indian subcontinent. Its development was a result of centuries of observations, experiments, and wisdom passed down through generations. Ayurveda's enduring appeal lies in its holistic and individualized approach to health, which continues to influence modern healthcare practices and lifestyles worldwide.

PRINCIPLES OF AYURVEDA SCIENCE

Ayurveda is an ancient system of medicine that originated in India. It is based on several fundamental principles:

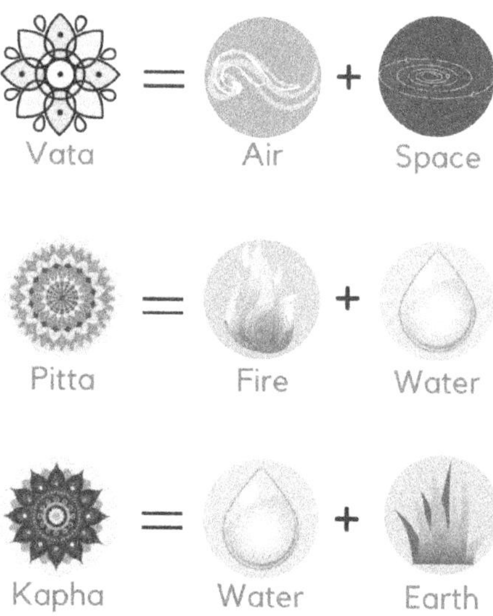

Fig: 2.2 Creation of Tridoshas from Panchmahabhut

Tridosha Theory: Ayurveda is founded on the concept of three doshas - Vata, Pitta, and Kapha. These doshas represent different combinations of the five elements (earth, water, fire, air, and ether) and are believed to govern various physiological and psychological functions in the body.

Panchamahabhutas: Ayurveda recognizes the five fundamental elements and their qualities, which play a significant role in the dosha constitution of an individual.

Prakriti (Constitution): Ayurveda holds that each person is born with a unique constitution (prakriti) determined by the predominance of doshas at birth. Understanding one's prakriti helps in maintaining health and preventing diseases.

Vikriti (Imbalance): Imbalance in the doshas from one's prakriti leads to illness. Ayurveda aims to identify these imbalances and restore harmony through various treatments and practices.

Sapta Dhatus: The human body is composed of seven primary tissues: Rasa (plasma), Rakta (blood), Mamsa (muscle), Meda (fat), Asthi (bone), Majja (marrow), and Shukra (reproductive tissues).

Agni (Digestive Fire): Proper digestion is central to good health in Ayurveda. Agni represents the body's digestive fire, and imbalances can lead to various health issues.

Malas: The body produces waste products (malas) such as urine, feces, and sweat. Their proper elimination is essential for maintaining health.

Srotas (Channels): Ayurveda believes in the existence of channels in the body through which nutrients, energy, and information flow. Keeping these channels clear is important for health.

Ama (Toxins): Incomplete digestion and metabolic waste can accumulate as ama in the body, leading to various diseases. Ayurvedic treatments aim to eliminate ama.

Rasayana and Vajikarana: These are rejuvenation and aphrodisiac therapies, respectively, aimed at promoting longevity and vitality.

Lifestyle and Diet: Ayurveda emphasizes the importance of a balanced lifestyle, including diet, exercise, and daily routines, to maintain health.

Herbal Medicine: Ayurveda makes extensive use of herbs and natural remedies to treat various conditions.

Yoga and Meditation: These practices are often recommended in Ayurveda to maintain physical and mental well-being.

Individualized Treatment: Ayurvedic treatments are personalized to an individual's constitution and imbalances.

It's important to note that Ayurveda is a holistic system that takes into accounts not only physical health but also mental, emotional, and spiritual well-being.

*****

Chapter 3

Ayurveda Market Analysis

समदोषः समाग्निश्च समधातुमलक्रियः ।

प्रसन्नात्मेन्द्रियमनाः स्वस्थ इत्यभिधीयते ॥४१॥

Samadosha Samagnishcha Sama Dhata Mala Kriya.
Prassanna atma indriya manah swastha iti abhideyate

An individual that maintains a balanced state of the main elements of the body (including *dosha* and *dhatu*), adequate digestion (*agni*), proper excretion (*mala kriya*), blissful condition of soul (*atma*), satisfied senses (*indriyan*) and a happy state of mind (*manas*) is called a*swasthya* or healthy person.

Sushruta Sutra, Chapter 15, verse 41

HIGHLIGHTS

Ayurveda's revival is driven by increased awareness, government support, modernization, alignment with global wellness trends.

Identifying niche areas and addressing market gaps in the Ayurvedic industry is essential for entrepreneurs to gain a competitive advantage, build consumer trust, promote sustainability, and enhance accessibility, ultimately contributing to the industry's growth.

CURRENT LOCAL AND GLOBAL TRENDS IN AYURVEDA

Ayurveda has seen resurgence in popularity in recent years, both locally and globally. This resurgence can be attributed to several current local and global trends.

Ayurvedic Market Size and Forecast

Ayurvedic Market size was valued at USD 6.50 Billion in 2020 and is projected to reach USD 21.12 Billion by 2028, growing at a CAGR of 15.63% from 2021 to 2028.

LOCAL TRENDS

Increased Awareness and Acceptance: In India, there has been a significant increase in awareness and acceptance of Ayurveda. Many people are now turning to Ayurveda for its holistic approach to healthcare and its emphasis on prevention.

Government Support: The Indian government has taken steps to promote Ayurveda. This includes setting up of Ministry of AYUSH, Ayurvedic research institutes, encouraging Ayurvedic education, and integrating Ayurveda into the national healthcare system.

Modernization of Ayurvedic Practices: Ayurvedic clinics and hospitals have modernized their practices. They have embraced technology for diagnosis, treatment, and record-keeping, making it more accessible and efficient.

Ayurveda in Wellness Tourism: India's wellness tourism industry has witnessed a surge, with many tourists seeking

Ayurvedic treatments, such as Panchakarma, yoga, and meditation, as part of their holistic wellness experiences.

GLOBAL TRENDS

GLOBAL AYURVEDA MARKET 2022-2026
Market growth will ACCELERATE at a CAGR of
15.32%
Growth Contributed by ASIA
79%
Incremental growth ($B)
6.81
2021
2026
Growth for 2022
14.64%
The market is FRAGMENTED with several players occupying the market
17000+ Reports covering niche topics. Read them at technavio

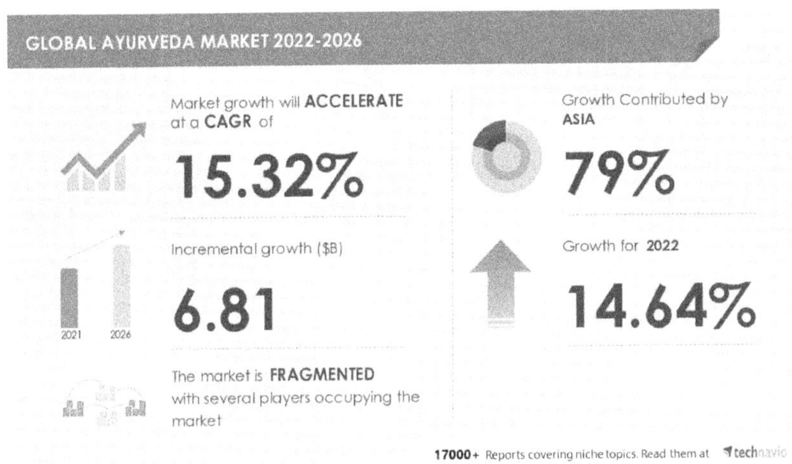

Fig: 3.1 Image showing global Ayurveda market growth

Holistic Health and Wellness: The global trend towards holistic health and wellness has boosted Ayurveda's popularity. People worldwide are seeking natural and holistic alternatives to conventional medicine.

Herbal and Plant-Based Medicine: Ayurveda's reliance on herbal remedies and plant-based medicine aligns with the global shift towards natural and sustainable healthcare options.

Personalized Medicine: Ayurveda's emphasis on individualized treatment plans based on one's dosha (constitution) aligns with the growing interest in personalized medicine and healthcare tailored to an individual's unique needs.

Yoga and Meditation: Ayurveda often goes hand in hand with practices like yoga and meditation, which have gained immense popularity worldwide for their physical and mental health benefits.

Scientific Validation: Ayurveda is increasingly subjected to scientific scrutiny, with researchers exploring its efficacy and safety. This trend enhances its credibility and acceptance on a global scale.

Global Ayurvedic Products Market: The demand for Ayurvedic products, including supplements, herbal cosmetics, and dietary items, is growing globally. Companies are capitalizing on this trend by offering Ayurvedic products to a wider audience.

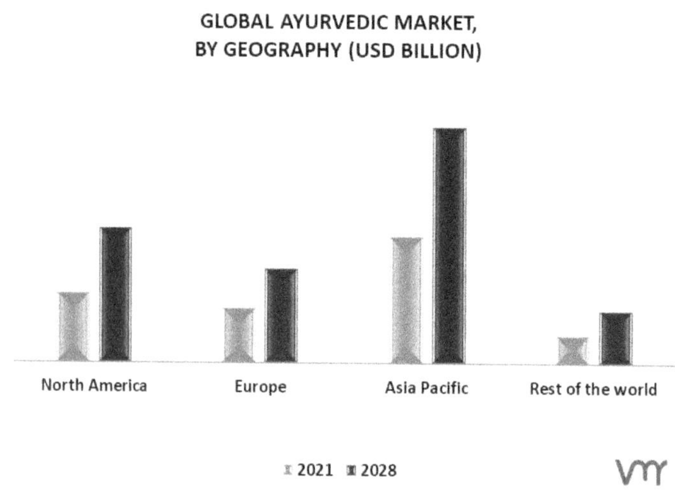

Fig: 3.2 Global Ayurveda product market by Geography

Conclusion: Ayurveda is experiencing a renaissance locally and globally due to a confluence of factors. Its focus on holistic health, personalized treatment, and natural remedies aligns with modern healthcare trends. With continued research and government support, Ayurveda is likely to maintain its relevance and further expand its reach in the future.

RISING DEMAND IN HOLISTIC WELLNESS

Holistic wellness, often referred to as holistic health or well-being, encompasses the idea that a person's health and happiness are a result of the harmonious balance between physical, mental, emotional, and spiritual aspects of life. It deviates from the conventional model of addressing only the physical symptoms of an ailment and instead seeks to understand the root causes of health issues.

One of the primary reasons for the increasing demand for holistic wellness is the recognition that traditional medical approaches sometimes fall short in providing comprehensive care. The limitations of Western medicine, such as overreliance on pharmaceuticals and a focus on symptom management rather than disease prevention, have led people to explore alternative options. Holistic wellness, with its focus on prevention and the integration of various healing practices, offers a more comprehensive approach to health.

The accessibility of information has played a vital role in the rise of holistic wellness. The internet and social media have made it easier for individuals to access a vast array of resources, from articles and videos to online courses and telehealth services. This has empowered people to take charge of their health and explore holistic wellness solutions that resonate with them.

Moreover, the stresses of modern life have prompted many to seek holistic approaches to managing mental and emotional well-being. Mindfulness practices, meditation, yoga, and other techniques have gained popularity as tools for stress reduction and emotional balance. These practices offer a way to address the root causes of emotional and mental health issues, rather than merely managing their symptoms.

Holistic wellness also aligns with a growing awareness of the importance of environmental and social well-being. People are increasingly recognizing the interconnectedness of all aspects of life and how they impact personal health. Sustainable living, ethical consumption, and community engagement are now seen as integral components of a holistic approach to wellness.

The rising demand for holistic wellness has far-reaching implications. It is reshaping the healthcare industry, with more healthcare providers integrating complementary and alternative therapies into their practices. It is also changing the way we view and approach well-being, emphasizing prevention and the importance of a healthy lifestyle. Society is gradually moving towards a more balanced and comprehensive approach to health, which could lead to better overall health outcomes and a higher quality of life for individuals.

In conclusion, the increasing demand for holistic wellness reflects a societal shift towards a more comprehensive and interconnected approach to health. As individuals seek solutions that address the physical, mental, emotional, and spiritual aspects of well-being, they are reshaping the healthcare landscape and promoting a holistic view of health that has the potential to benefit individuals and society as a whole.

IDENTIFYING NICHE AREAS AND MARKET GAPS FOR NEW VENTURES IN AYURVEDA

This revival has created a plethora of opportunities for entrepreneurs to establish new ventures in the Ayurvedic industry. To succeed in this highly competitive market, it is essential to identify niche areas and market gaps. This essay will explore strategies to pinpoint these opportunities and discuss the importance of addressing unmet needs in the Ayurvedic sector.

UNDERSTANDING THE AYURVEDA MARKET

Before delving into niche areas and market gaps, one must comprehend the current state of the Ayurvedic market. The global wellness industry, of which Ayurveda is a significant part, has been expanding steadily due to increasing health awareness and a preference for natural remedies. In this context, Ayurveda offers a holistic approach, emphasizing personalized wellness plans based on individual body types or "Doshas."

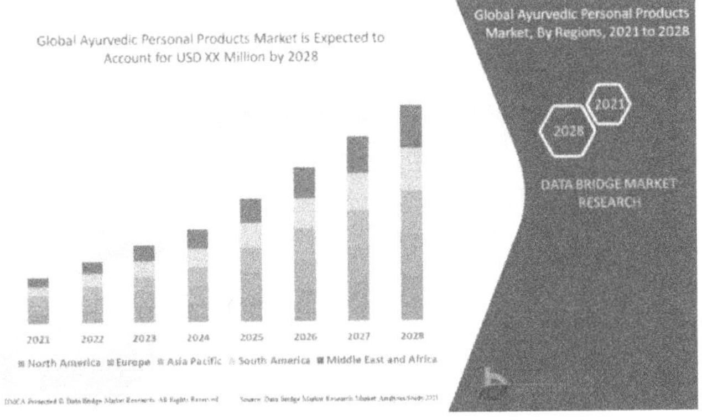

Fig: 3.3 Image showing global ayurvedic personal product market

IDENTIFYING NICHE AREAS

Personalized Ayurvedic Solutions: Tailoring Ayurvedic treatments and products to individual Doshas is an emerging trend. Entrepreneurs can specialize in creating personalized herbal formulations and wellness plans for consumers based on their unique constitutions.

Herbal Supplements and Nutraceuticals: The demand for Ayurvedic herbal supplements and nutraceuticals is on the rise. Entrepreneurs can focus on producing high-quality, standardized herbal products that cater to specific health needs, such as stress management, immunity boosting, or skin care.

Ayurveda in Beauty and Skincare: Ayurvedic beauty and skincare products are gaining popularity. Entrepreneurs can explore the development of organic, Ayurvedic cosmetics and skincare lines, addressing the demand for natural and sustainable alternatives.

Ayurveda Tourism: Wellness tourism, with a strong emphasis on Ayurveda, is a growing sector. Entrepreneurs can establish retreat centers, spas, or wellness resorts that offer authentic Ayurvedic treatments and experiences.

IDENTIFYING MARKET GAPS

Certification and Quality Assurance: Ensuring the authenticity and quality of Ayurvedic products is a significant challenge. Entrepreneurs can develop third-party certification services or quality assurance mechanisms to address this gap.

Digital Health Platforms: Ayurvedic consultation and treatment delivery through digital platforms are an unexplored territory. Entrepreneurs can create user-friendly apps or platforms that connect Ayurvedic practitioners with patients, enhancing accessibility and convenience.

Research and Education: The lack of standardized education and research in Ayurveda creates a gap. Entrepreneurs can establish Ayurvedic schools, research institutions, or online platforms that promote knowledge exchange and collaboration.

Sustainable Sourcing and Packaging: Sustainable sourcing of herbs and eco-friendly packaging are areas where the Ayurvedic industry can improve. Entrepreneurs can focus on environmentally friendly practices to address this concern.

IMPORTANCE OF ADDRESSING MARKET GAPS

Identifying and addressing market gaps in the Ayurvedic industry is crucial for several reasons:

Competitive Advantage: Meeting unmet needs provides a competitive advantage and can help new ventures stand out in a crowded market.

Consumer Trust: By offering solutions to issues like authenticity and quality, entrepreneurs can build trust with consumers, enhancing their brand reputation.

Sustainability: Addressing gaps in sustainable sourcing and packaging contributes to the long-term viability of Ayurvedic ventures in an environmentally conscious world.

Access and Convenience: Bridging gaps in education and digital health platforms can make Ayurvedic knowledge and services more accessible to a global audience.

Conclusion: In the dynamic landscape of the Ayurvedic industry, identifying niche areas and market gaps is a fundamental step for entrepreneurs looking to establish successful ventures. The combination of personalized solutions, product innovation, and addressing issues of quality, education, and sustainability will not only enable growth but also contribute to the broader adoption of Ayurveda as a holistic and sustainable approach to wellness. Entrepreneurs who can successfully identify and address these areas of opportunity are well-positioned to thrive in this flourishing industry.

*****

Section-2

Exploring Ayurveda Business Opportunities

Chapter 4

Ayurveda Hospitals and Clinics

प्रयोगज्ञानविज्ञानसिद्धिसिद्धाः सुखप्रदाः|
जीविताभिसरास्ते स्युर्वैद्यत्वं तेष्ववस्थितमिति||५३||

Prayoggyanvighyansidhisidhah sukhpradah,
jivitabhisraaste syurvaidhyatvam teshvavasthitamiti

Those who are accomplished in the administration of therapies, insight, and knowledge of therapeutics, are endowed with infallible success and can bring happiness to the seeker. They are saviors of life.

Charaka Sutra Sthana,Chapter 11, verse 53

HIGHLIGHTS

The establishment of a state-of-the-art Ayurveda hospital combines traditional Ayurvedic wisdom with modern healthcare, resulting in holistic patient care, better health outcomes, cultural preservation, and economic growth.

The takeaway is that Single Specialty Ayurveda Clinics are better because they offer specialized, personalized, and comprehensive care for specific health concerns, bridging traditional and modern medicine to promote holistic well-being.

STATE OF THE ART AYURVEDA HOSPITAL

Establishing a state-of-the-art Ayurveda hospital represents a significant step in promoting traditional healing methods while integrating modern technology and standards of healthcare. This essay explores the key aspects of setting up such a hospital, its importance, and the potential benefits it can offer to the community.

THE NEED FOR A STATE-OF-THE-ART AYURVEDA HOSPITAL

Preserving Traditional Knowledge: Ayurveda is deeply rooted in ancient Indian wisdom, with a rich history spanning thousands of years. By establishing a state-of-the-art Ayurveda hospital, we can help preserve and promote this traditional knowledge.

Holistic Healthcare: Ayurveda focuses on holistic wellness, considering the mind, body, and spirit as interconnected. Such an approach can provide a more comprehensive and patient-centered healthcare experience.

Integrating Modern Technology: Incorporating modern medical technology and infrastructure into an Ayurveda hospital ensures safety, efficiency, and precision in diagnosis and treatment, improving the overall quality of care.

Meeting Growing Demand: With the growing interest in alternative and complementary medicine, there is a rising demand for Ayurvedic treatments. A state-of-the-art Ayurveda hospital can cater to this demand effectively.

KEY COMPONENTS OF A STATE-OF-THE-ART AYURVEDA HOSPITAL

Experienced Practitioners: The cornerstone of any Ayurveda hospital is a team of experienced and skilled Ayurvedic practitioners who can provide personalized care to patients.

Research and Development: Investing in research to validate the efficacy of Ayurvedic treatments and develop new therapies is essential for the hospital's success.

Modern Infrastructure: The hospital should be equipped with state-of-the-art facilities, including diagnostic equipment, patient rooms, and treatment centers, to ensure the highest standards of healthcare.

Accreditation and Certification: Obtaining the necessary certifications and accreditations is crucial to build trust and confidence among patients and the medical community.

Patient Education: Educating patients about Ayurveda and its benefits is a vital part of the hospital's mission. Workshops, seminars, and information dissemination play a role in empowering individuals to make informed healthcare choices.

BENEFITS OF A STATE-OF-THE-ART AYURVEDA HOSPITAL

Comprehensive Care: Patients can receive integrated care that combines the strengths of Ayurveda and modern medicine for a well-rounded approach to healing.

Improved Patient Outcomes: By leveraging modern technology and research, Ayurveda can deliver even better results, addressing chronic illnesses and enhancing overall wellness.

Cultural Preservation: The hospital can contribute to the preservation of India's rich cultural heritage by promoting and nurturing Ayurvedic traditions.

Economic Growth: Establishing a state-of-the-art Ayurveda hospital can stimulate economic growth by creating jobs and promoting medical tourism.

Conclusion: The establishment of a state-of-the-art Ayurveda hospital serves as a bridge between the ancient wisdom of Ayurveda and the demands of modern healthcare. By combining traditional knowledge with modern advancements, such a hospital can provide holistic and effective healthcare while preserving the heritage of Ayurveda. It's a step toward a healthier, more informed, and culturally rich future for both the local community and the global population seeking alternative healthcare options.

SINGLE SPECIALTY AYURVEDA CLINICS

Expertise and Specialization: Single Specialty Ayurveda Clinics allow practitioners to specialize and gain expertise in specific areas of Ayurveda. This specialization enables them to provide more focused and effective treatments for patients suffering from particular ailments or conditions. For example, clinics specializing in Panchakarma can offer in-depth detoxification and rejuvenation therapies.

Tailored Treatments: Each Ayurvedic specialty clinic is designed to cater to a particular health concern, which means treatments and therapies are tailored to address those concerns. Patients can expect personalized care that aligns with their specific needs, enhancing the effectiveness of Ayurvedic treatments.

Comprehensive Care: Specialty Ayurveda clinics often provide comprehensive care by combining traditional Ayurvedic methods with modern medical practices. This integration can improve patient outcomes and offer a more holistic approach to healthcare.

TYPES OF SPECIALTY AYURVEDA CLINICS

PANCHAKARMA CLINICS

Panchakarma is a traditional Ayurvedic therapy that has been practiced for centuries in India. Panchakarma clinics are specialized centers where individuals can undergo this therapeutic process to detoxify and rejuvenate their bodies. These clinics offer a comprehensive and holistic approach to wellness, focusing on the physical, mental, and spiritual aspects of health.

The Essence of Panchakarma: Panchakarma, which means "five actions" in Sanskrit, is a set of purification and rejuvenation techniques designed to balance the body's doshas (Vata, Pitta, and Kapha) and eliminate toxins. The five primary actions of Panchakarma include Vamana (emesis), Virechana (purgation), Basti (enema), Nasya (nasal therapy), and Raktamokshana (bloodletting). These therapies are tailored to an individual's constitution and specific health concerns.

KEY COMPONENTS OF A PANCHAKARMA CLINIC

Experienced Ayurvedic Practitioners: Panchakarma clinics are staffed with skilled Ayurvedic practitioners who assess each patient's unique constitution, health history, and current imbalances. This personalized approach ensures that the Panchakarma therapies are tailored to the individual's needs.

Detoxification and Rejuvenation: The core objective of Panchakarma is to remove accumulated toxins from the body, promoting better health and vitality. This process involves a sequence of therapies, each focusing on specific detoxification mechanisms.

Dietary Guidance: Panchakarma clinics provide dietary recommendations that support the detoxification process and help maintain balance after treatment. Ayurvedic nutrition plays a crucial role in this regard, with an emphasis on wholesome, individualized diets.

Yoga and Meditation: Many Panchakarma clinics incorporate yoga and meditation practices to address the mental and spiritual dimensions of health. These techniques enhance relaxation, reduce stress, and promote overall well-being.

Herbal Medicines: Herbal remedies, formulated according to Ayurvedic principles, are often prescribed during and after Panchakarma treatment to support the body's healing process and maintain balance.

Lifestyle Counseling: Panchakarma clinics offer guidance on lifestyle adjustments that are in harmony with Ayurvedic principles. These recommendations can include daily routines, exercise, and stress management techniques.

Benefits of Panchakarma: Panchakarma offers numerous benefits, including:

Detoxification: Eliminating accumulated toxins and waste from the body.

Improved Digestion: Enhancing digestive function and metabolism.

Stress Reduction: Reducing stress and promoting mental clarity.

Enhanced Immunity: Strengthening the immune system.

Chronic Disease Management: Managing chronic health conditions like arthritis, digestive disorders, and skin issues.

Conclusion: Panchakarma clinics provide a holistic approach to wellness by combining traditional Ayurvedic therapies, personalized care, and a focus on physical, mental, and spiritual well-being. This ancient practice has found relevance in modern times as people seek natural and comprehensive methods to maintain and restore their health. Panchakarma clinics are hubs of holistic healing that continue to promote balance, detoxification, and rejuvenation for individuals in pursuit of optimal well-being.

AYURVEDA DERMATOLOGY CLINICS

The Ayurveda Dermatology Clinic represents a harmonious blend of ancient Ayurvedic wisdom and modern dermatological science. It is a specialized healthcare facility where individuals can seek solutions for skin, hair, and nail-related issues while benefiting from the holistic principles of Ayurveda. This essay explores the key components and advantages of an Ayurveda Dermatology Clinic.

Foundations of Ayurveda Dermatology: Ayurveda, an ancient system of medicine originating in India, places a strong emphasis on understanding the body's constitution (Prakriti), the balance of doshas (Vata, Pitta, Kapha), and the impact of these factors on overall health. Ayurvedic dermatology is an extension of this philosophy, recognizing the intimate connection between skin health and internal imbalances.

KEY COMPONENTS OF AN AYURVEDA DERMATOLOGY CLINIC

Ayurvedic Expertise: At the heart of these clinics are Ayurvedic practitioners who are trained to diagnose skin conditions not only from a conventional dermatological standpoint but also through Ayurvedic principles. They consider doshic imbalances, digestion, lifestyle, and emotional factors that may contribute to skin issues.

Herbal Therapies: One of the cornerstones of Ayurveda Dermatology is the use of herbal remedies and formulations to address skin disorders. These natural treatments are customized to suit the unique constitution and specific skin concerns of each patient.

Diet and Lifestyle Counseling: Clinics often provide guidance on dietary modifications and lifestyle changes tailored to an individual's constitution. Such adjustments help restore balance and improve skin health from within.

Panchakarma for Skin: Panchakarma, a traditional Ayurvedic detoxification and rejuvenation therapy, can be used to treat skin issues. Procedures like Abhyanga (oil massage) and Swedana (sweating therapy) can help alleviate skin conditions by purifying the body.

Holistic Skin Care: Ayurvedic skin care is holistic, focusing on the use of natural ingredients, avoidance of harmful chemicals, and the incorporation of self-care practices. It promotes long-term skin health and beauty.

BENEFITS OF AYURVEDA DERMATOLOGY CLINICS

Holistic Approach: These clinics address skin problems at their root, considering the whole person, including mental and physical aspects, rather than merely offering topical solutions.

Personalization: Treatments are tailored to the individual's Prakriti, ensuring the best possible outcomes.

Minimal Side Effects: Ayurvedic treatments are generally safe with minimal side effects, making them suitable for a wide range of patients.

Chronic Skin Conditions: Ayurveda Dermatology can effectively manage chronic skin conditions like eczema, psoriasis, and acne, providing relief and improved quality of life.

Conclusion: The Ayurveda Dermatology Clinic represents a bridge between traditional Ayurvedic wisdom and modern dermatological science. It offers a holistic approach to skin health, emphasizing individualized care, natural remedies, and a deep understanding of the interconnectedness of skin and overall well-being. In an era where the demand for natural and personalized skin care solutions is growing, Ayurveda Dermatology Clinics provide a unique and effective approach to address a wide array of skin conditions while promoting long-term skin health and vitality.

AYURVEDA TRICHOLOGY CLINICS

The Ayurveda Trichology Clinic is a specialized healthcare facility that combines the principles of Ayurveda and trichology to address various hair and scalp-related issues. Trichology is the branch of dermatology that focuses on the study of hair and scalp health. This essay explores the key components and benefits of an Ayurveda Trichology Clinic, where traditional Ayurvedic practices are integrated with modern hair care science.

The Intersection of Ayurveda and Trichology: Ayurveda, an ancient Indian system of medicine, emphasizes a holistic approach to health, considering an individual's unique constitution (Prakriti), doshic imbalances (Vata, Pitta, Kapha), and the impact of these factors on overall well-being. Trichology, on the other hand, is a contemporary field that specializes in diagnosing and treating hair and scalp disorders using scientific methods. The Ayurveda Trichology Clinic brings these two worlds together to offer comprehensive solutions for hair and scalp health.

KEY COMPONENTS OF AN AYURVEDA TRICHOLOGY CLINIC

Ayurvedic Trichologists: The clinic is staffed with Ayurvedic trichologists who are experts in both Ayurveda and trichology. They utilize their knowledge to diagnose hair and scalp issues through an Ayurvedic lens and modern scientific techniques.

Hair and Scalp Analysis: Advanced tools and methods are used for in-depth analysis of hair and scalp conditions. This may include hair microscopy, digital imaging, and laboratory tests to identify the root causes of hair problems.

Herbal Treatments: Herbal remedies and formulations are central to Ayurvedic trichology. These natural treatments are personalized for each patient, addressing specific hair and scalp concerns while considering their unique constitution.

Lifestyle and Dietary Guidance: The clinic provides recommendations for dietary adjustments and lifestyle modifications based on Ayurvedic principles. This holistic approach helps balance internal factors that can affect hair health.

Panchakarma for Hair: Panchakarma, an Ayurvedic detoxification and rejuvenation therapy, is adapted for trichology. Procedures like Shirodhara (oil pouring on the head) and Nasya (nasal therapy) can be employed to improve scalp and hair health.

BENEFITS OF AYURVEDA TRICHOLOGY CLINICS

Personalized Care: Treatments are customized according to an individual's Prakriti, ensuring a more effective approach to hair and scalp concerns.

Natural Solutions: Ayurvedic treatments are based on natural ingredients and are free from harmful chemicals, making them suitable for a wide range of patients.

Minimal Side Effects: The treatments generally have minimal side effects, making them safer than some conventional hair care options.

Effective Management: Ayurvedic trichology can effectively manage various hair problems such as hair loss, dandruff, premature graying, and alopecia.

Conclusion: The Ayurveda Trichology Clinic is a unique and comprehensive center for addressing hair and scalp issues through the lens of both Ayurveda and trichology. It offers a holistic approach to hair care, emphasizing individualized and natural solutions for healthier hair and scalp. In a time when people seek alternatives to chemical-laden hair treatments, Ayurveda Trichology Clinics provide a bridge between ancient wisdom and modern science, focusing on long-term hair health and vitality.

AYURVEDA ORTHOPEDIC CLINICS

The Ayurveda Orthopedic Clinic represents a unique healthcare facility that blends the ancient wisdom of Ayurveda with modern orthopedic practices to treat musculoskeletal conditions. Ayurveda, a holistic Indian system of medicine, addresses the root causes of health issues, while orthopedics focuses on the diagnosis and treatment of musculoskeletal disorders. This essay explores the key components and benefits of an Ayurveda Orthopedic Clinic, where these two disciplines come together to offer comprehensive solutions for orthopedic patients.

The Fusion of Ayurveda and Orthopedics: Ayurveda places significant emphasis on understanding an individual's constitution (Prakriti), doshic imbalances (Vata, Pitta, Kapha), and the impact of these factors on health. Orthopedics, on the other hand, specializes in the diagnosis and treatment of conditions affecting the musculoskeletal system, including bones, joints, muscles, and ligaments. The Ayurveda Orthopedic Clinic bridges these two worlds to provide patients with a holistic approach to musculoskeletal health.

KEY COMPONENTS OF AN AYURVEDA ORTHOPEDIC CLINIC

Ayurvedic Orthopedic Specialists: The clinic is staffed with experts who are well-versed in both Ayurveda and orthopedics. These specialists use Ayurvedic principles to understand the underlying imbalances contributing to musculoskeletal issues.

Diagnosis and Assessment: Advanced diagnostic tools, including X-rays, MRIs, and other imaging techniques, are utilized to accurately diagnose musculoskeletal conditions. Ayurvedic assessments are integrated to provide a holistic view of the patient's health.

Herbal Remedies: Ayurvedic herbal treatments and formulations are central to the clinic's approach. These natural therapies are customized to address the specific musculoskeletal concerns of each patient while considering their unique constitution.

Lifestyle and Dietary Guidance: The clinic provides recommendations for lifestyle modifications and dietary changes based on Ayurvedic principles. These adjustments help restore balance and promote overall well-being, which is crucial for musculoskeletal health.

Panchakarma for Orthopedics: Panchakarma, an Ayurvedic detoxification and rejuvenation therapy, is adapted for orthopedic patients. Procedures like Abhyanga (oil massage) and Swedana (sweating therapy) can be employed to improve musculoskeletal health.

BENEFITS OF AYURVEDA ORTHOPEDIC CLINICS

Holistic Care: These clinics offer a more comprehensive approach to musculoskeletal issues by addressing the root causes and promoting overall health.

Personalized Treatments: Ayurvedic treatments are tailored to an individual's Prakriti, ensuring a more effective approach to orthopedic concerns.

Natural Solutions: Ayurvedic remedies are based on natural ingredients and are generally free from harmful chemicals, making them suitable for a wide range of patients.

Effective Management: Ayurveda Orthopedic Clinics can effectively manage musculoskeletal conditions such as arthritis, back pain, joint issues, and sports injuries.

Conclusion: The Ayurveda Orthopedic Clinic is a unique and valuable resource for individuals seeking holistic solutions for musculoskeletal issues. By combining the principles of Ayurveda and modern orthopedic care, these clinics offer a bridge between ancient wisdom and contemporary medical science. In an era where many patients seek natural and individualized approaches to orthopedic concerns, Ayurveda Orthopedic Clinics provide a comprehensive strategy for restoring musculoskeletal health, promoting well-being, and managing conditions more effectively.

AYURVEDA GYNAECOLOGY CLINICS

The Ayurveda Gynaecology Clinic is a specialized healthcare facility dedicated to addressing women's health concerns using the principles of Ayurveda. Ayurveda, an ancient Indian system of medicine, emphasizes a holistic approach to health and wellness. In the context of gynaecology, Ayurveda offers unique insights and natural treatments for a wide range of women's health issues. This essay explores the key components and advantages of an Ayurveda Gynaecology Clinic, where traditional Ayurvedic practices are integrated with modern gynaecological care.

The Intersection of Ayurveda and Gynaecology: Ayurveda recognizes the unique physiological and emotional aspects of women's health and provides an integrated approach to gynaecology. It takes into consideration an individual's constitution (Prakriti), doshic imbalances (Vata, Pitta, Kapha), and the impact of these factors on women's health. By combining the wisdom of Ayurveda with gynaecological expertise, the Ayurveda Gynaecology Clinic offers a holistic approach to women's well-being.

KEY COMPONENTS OF AN AYURVEDA GYNAECOLOGY CLINIC

Ayurvedic Gynaecologists: The clinic is staffed with Ayurvedic gynaecologists who are experts in both Ayurveda and women's health. They use Ayurvedic principles to diagnose and treat gynaecological conditions, including menstrual disorders, fertility issues, and menopausal symptoms.

Herbal Therapies: Herbal remedies and formulations are central to the clinic's approach. These natural treatments are personalized for each patient, addressing specific gynaecological concerns while considering their unique constitution.

Dietary and Lifestyle Guidance: The clinic provides recommendations for dietary adjustments and lifestyle modifications based on Ayurvedic principles. These adjustments help balance internal factors that can affect women's health, such as hormonal imbalances.

Panchakarma for Women: Panchakarma, an Ayurvedic detoxification and rejuvenation therapy, is adapted for women's health. Procedures like Abhyanga (oil massage) and Yoni Pichu (vaginal oil therapy) can be employed to improve gynaecological well-being.

Holistic Women's Health Care: The clinic offers holistic women's health care, which includes the promotion of mental and emotional well-being. Techniques such as yoga and meditation are often integrated into treatment plans.

BENEFITS OF AYURVEDA GYNAECOLOGY CLINICS

Holistic Care: These clinics offer a more comprehensive approach to women's health by addressing the root causes of gynaecological issues and promoting overall well-being.

Personalized Treatments: Ayurvedic treatments are tailored to an individual's Prakriti, ensuring a more effective approach to gynaecological concerns.

Natural Solutions: Ayurvedic remedies are based on natural ingredients and are generally free from harmful chemicals, making them suitable for a wide range of patients.

Effective Management: Ayurveda Gynaecology Clinics can effectively manage conditions such as menstrual irregularities, polycystic ovarian syndrome (PCOS), and menopausal symptoms.

Conclusion: The Ayurveda Gynaecology Clinic serves as a bridge between traditional Ayurvedic wisdom and modern gynaecological care. It offers a holistic approach to women's health, emphasizing individualized and natural solutions for a wide range of gynaecological concerns. In an era where women increasingly seek natural and personalized approaches to women's health, Ayurveda Gynaecology Clinics provide a comprehensive strategy for promoting and maintaining women's well-being throughout their life stages.

AYURVEDA MENTAL HEALTH CLINICS

The Ayurveda Mental Health Clinic is a specialized healthcare facility that marries the ancient principles of Ayurveda with contemporary mental health care. Ayurveda, a traditional Indian system of medicine, focuses on the holistic well-being of individuals. In the context of mental health, Ayurveda offers a unique approach to understanding and addressing psychological issues. This essay explores the key components and advantages of an Ayurveda Mental Health Clinic, where traditional Ayurvedic practices are integrated with modern mental health care.

The Intersection of Ayurveda and Mental Health: Ayurveda recognizes the intricate connection between the mind and body and considers the doshas (Vata, Pitta, Kapha) when assessing an individual's mental health. Mental well-being is seen as a reflection of the balance and harmony of these doshas, as well as the state of the mind. By combining the wisdom of Ayurveda with modern psychology and psychiatry, Ayurveda Mental Health Clinics provide a holistic approach to mental health.

KEY COMPONENTS OF AN AYURVEDA MENTAL HEALTH CLINIC

Ayurvedic Mental Health Specialists: The clinic is staffed with professionals who are experts in both Ayurveda and mental health. These specialists use Ayurvedic principles to diagnose and treat mental health conditions, including stress, anxiety, depression, and mood disorders.

Herbal Therapies: Herbal remedies and formulations are central to the clinic's approach. These natural treatments are personalized for each patient, addressing specific mental health concerns while considering their unique constitution.

Dietary and Lifestyle Guidance: The clinic provides recommendations for dietary adjustments and lifestyle modifications based on Ayurvedic principles. These adjustments help balance internal factors that can affect mental well-being, including diet and daily routines.

Panchakarma for Mental Health: Panchakarma, an Ayurvedic detoxification and rejuvenation therapy, is adapted for mental health. Procedures like Shirodhara (oil pouring on the head) and Nasya (nasal therapy) can be employed to improve mental well-being and reduce stress.

Holistic Mental Health Care: The clinic offers holistic mental health care that emphasizes not only psychological well-being but also emotional and spiritual balance. Techniques such as yoga and meditation are often integrated into treatment plans.

BENEFITS OF AYURVEDA MENTAL HEALTH CLINICS

Holistic Care: These clinics offer a more comprehensive approach to mental health by addressing the root causes of psychological issues and promoting overall well-being.

Personalized Treatments: Ayurvedic treatments are tailored to an individual's constitution (Prakriti) and doshic imbalances, ensuring a more effective approach to mental health concerns.

Natural Solutions: Ayurvedic remedies are based on natural ingredients and are generally free from harmful chemicals, making them suitable for a wide range of patients.

Effective Management: Ayurveda Mental Health Clinics can effectively manage mental health conditions, providing relief and improved quality of life for those suffering from stress, anxiety, depression, and related disorders.

Conclusion: The Ayurveda Mental Health Clinic serves as a bridge between traditional Ayurvedic wisdom and modern mental health care. It offers a holistic approach to mental health, emphasizing individualized and natural solutions for a wide range of psychological concerns. In an era where individuals seek natural and personalized approaches to mental health, Ayurveda Mental Health Clinics provide a comprehensive strategy for promoting and maintaining psychological well-being and harmony in the modern world.

AYURVEDA DIGESTIVE HEALTH CLINICS

The Ayurveda Digestive Health Clinic is a specialized healthcare facility that blends the profound insights of Ayurveda with modern digestive health practices. Ayurveda, a traditional Indian system of medicine, emphasizes holistic wellness and considers the digestive system as the foundation of overall health. This essay delves into the key components and benefits of an Ayurveda Digestive Health Clinic, where ancient Ayurvedic principles are harmoniously integrated with contemporary digestive care.

The Marriage of Ayurveda and Digestive Health: Ayurveda recognizes the critical role of digestion in maintaining overall health and well-being. It assesses an individual's constitution (Prakriti), doshic imbalances (Vata, Pitta, Kapha), and dietary habits to understand and address digestive issues. By combining the wisdom of Ayurveda with modern digestive care, the Ayurveda Digestive Health Clinic offers a holistic approach to digestive well-being.

KEY COMPONENTS OF AN AYURVEDA DIGESTIVE HEALTH CLINIC

Ayurvedic Digestive Health Specialists: The clinic employs professionals well-versed in both Ayurveda and digestive health. These experts use Ayurvedic principles to diagnose and treat digestive disorders, including irritable bowel syndrome (IBS), acid reflux, and food sensitivities.

Herbal Remedies: Herbal treatments and formulations are central to the clinic's approach. These natural therapies are tailored for each patient, addressing specific digestive concerns while considering their unique constitution and doshic imbalances.

Dietary and Lifestyle Guidance: The clinic provides recommendations for dietary adjustments and lifestyle modifications based on Ayurvedic principles. These changes help restore balance and promote overall well-being, particularly with regard to digestive health.

Panchakarma for Digestive Health: Panchakarma, an Ayurvedic detoxification and rejuvenation therapy, is adapted for digestive health. Procedures like Virechana (purgation) and Basti (enema) can be employed to cleanse and revitalize the digestive system.

Holistic Digestive Wellness: The clinic emphasizes holistic digestive health, incorporating mindfulness techniques, stress management, and yoga to promote mental and emotional well-being alongside physical wellness.

BENEFITS OF AYURVEDA DIGESTIVE HEALTH CLINICS

Comprehensive Care: These clinics offer a more comprehensive approach to digestive health by addressing the root causes of digestive issues and promoting overall well-being.

Personalized Treatments: Ayurvedic treatments are tailored to an individual's constitution and doshic imbalances, ensuring a more effective approach to digestive concerns.

Natural Solutions: Ayurvedic remedies are based on natural ingredients and are typically free from harmful chemicals, making them suitable for a wide range of patients.

Effective Management: Ayurveda Digestive Health Clinics can effectively manage digestive conditions, providing relief for individuals dealing with a range of issues, from indigestion to chronic gastrointestinal disorders.

Conclusion: The Ayurveda Digestive Health Clinic acts as a bridge between traditional Ayurvedic wisdom and modern digestive health care. It offers a holistic approach to digestive well-being, emphasizing individualized and natural solutions for various digestive concerns. In a world where individuals are increasingly seeking natural and personalized approaches to digestive health, Ayurveda Digestive Health Clinics provide a comprehensive strategy for promoting and maintaining digestive wellness, vital for overall health and vitality

AYURVEDIC WEIGHT MANAGEMENT CLINICS

Ayurveda, one of the world's oldest holistic healing systems, has gained significant recognition for its natural and holistic approach to weight management. Ayurvedic weight management clinics offer individuals a unique blend of ancient wisdom and modern science to address the rising concern of obesity and its related health issues. This essay explores the principles, treatments, and benefits of Ayurvedic weight management clinics.

THE PRINCIPLES OF AYURVEDIC WEIGHT MANAGEMENT

Individual Constitution (Prakriti): Ayurveda identifies three main body types, or doshas (Vata, Pitta, and Kapha). Each person has a unique constitution, and Ayurvedic weight management considers the individual's dosha when devising a personalized plan.

Balance of Doshas: The imbalance of doshas is often at the root of weight gain. Ayurvedic practitioners aim to restore this balance through dietary and lifestyle changes, along with herbal remedies.

Mind-Body Connection: Ayurveda recognizes the strong connection between mental and physical health. Stress, emotional imbalances, and poor lifestyle choices can lead to weight gain. Ayurvedic treatments address these factors.

TREATMENTS OFFERED IN AYURVEDIC WEIGHT MANAGEMENT CLINICS

Dietary Guidance: Ayurvedic experts prescribe personalized diets that align with an individual's dosha. This often includes a focus on whole, unprocessed foods and mindful eating practices.

Herbal Supplements: Natural herbs and remedies are used to support metabolism, digestion, and detoxification. These are carefully chosen to suit the person's constitution.

Lifestyle Modifications: Ayurvedic clinics emphasize the importance of daily routines (dinacharya) and seasonal routines (ritucharya) to promote wellness. These routines can include exercise, yoga, meditation, and adequate sleep.

Detoxification (Panchakarma): Panchakarma is a detoxification process that includes therapies like oil massages, herbal steam baths, and cleansing enemas. It helps remove toxins from the body and balance the doshas.

BENEFITS OF AYURVEDIC WEIGHT MANAGEMENT CLINICS

Sustainable Weight Loss: Ayurveda focuses on long-term lifestyle changes rather than quick fixes, making weight loss more sustainable.

Holistic Health Improvement: Ayurvedic treatments not only help with weight management but also enhance overall well-being by addressing the root causes of health issues.

Personalized Approach: By considering an individual's constitution, Ayurvedic clinics provide customized solutions, which can be more effective than one-size-fits-all approaches.

Natural and Safe: Ayurvedic treatments primarily rely on natural herbs and therapies, minimizing the risk of side effects often associated with pharmaceutical interventions.

Stress Reduction: Ayurveda emphasizes stress management, which can be a significant factor in weight gain. Stress reduction techniques lead to better mental health.

Conclusion: Ayurvedic weight management clinics offer a holistic and time-tested approach to weight management that prioritizes individualized care and overall well-being. While Ayurveda's effectiveness may vary from person to person, it provides an alternative path for those seeking a natural, balanced, and sustainable approach to weight loss and improved health. As the world grapples with the challenges of obesity and its related health problems, Ayurvedic weight management clinics stand as an ancient yet relevant solution.

AYURVEDA BEAUTY CLINICS

In the pursuit of beauty and well-being, many individuals are turning to Ayurveda Beauty Clinics as a holistic alternative to conventional beauty treatments. Ayurveda, an ancient system of medicine originating in India, places a strong emphasis on the interconnectedness of mind, body, and spirit. Ayurveda Beauty Clinics offer a unique approach to beauty that goes beyond superficial treatments and focuses on promoting overall health and balance. This essay explores the concept of Ayurveda Beauty Clinics, their principles, services, and the benefits they offer.

SERVICES OFFERED BY AYURVEDA BEAUTY CLINICS

Ayurveda Beauty Clinics provide a range of services that align with the principles of Ayurveda. These services are designed to restore balance and enhance an individual's natural beauty. Some common services offered include:

Ayurvedic Skin Care: Customized skincare treatments that use natural ingredients and herbal formulations to address skin issues and promote a healthy complexion.

Ayurvedic Hair Care: Hair treatments that focus on nourishing the scalp and hair, using herbs and oils to maintain healthy and lustrous locks.

Ayurvedic Massages: Therapeutic massages that use herbal oils to relax the body, reduce stress, and improve circulation, which indirectly enhances the skin's radiance.

Diet and Nutrition: Ayurvedic clinics often provide dietary recommendations based on an individual's dosha, ensuring that nutrition supports overall health and beauty.

Stress Reduction: Stress management techniques, including yoga and meditation, to achieve mental peace and emotional balance, which are considered essential for beauty.

BENEFITS OF AYURVEDA BEAUTY CLINICS

The Ayurveda Beauty Clinic approach to beauty offers several benefits:

Natural and Safe: Ayurvedic treatments rely on natural ingredients and holistic approaches, minimizing the use of chemicals and synthetic products that may have adverse effects on the skin and body.

Balanced Beauty: Rather than focusing solely on superficial aspects, Ayurveda Beauty Clinics address the root causes of beauty issues by promoting balance and well-being.

Customization: Treatments are personalized based on an individual's dosha and specific needs, ensuring that they are effective and harmonious.

Long-Lasting Results: Ayurvedic beauty treatments aim for lasting results by addressing the underlying imbalances in the body.

Stress Reduction: The incorporation of stress-reduction techniques improves mental well-being, which is closely linked to an individual's appearance.

Conclusion: Ayurveda Beauty Clinics represent a holistic and well-rounded approach to beauty and well-being. In a world where cosmetic enhancements and quick fixes are prevalent, Ayurveda offers an alternative that focuses on long-term health and balanced beauty. By embracing the principles of Ayurveda and the services provided by these clinics, individuals can find an avenue to enhance their natural beauty while promoting physical and mental harmony. In essence, Ayurveda Beauty Clinics are a reflection of the age-old wisdom that true beauty radiates from the inside out.

AYURVEDA SPA AND WELLNESS CENTRE

Ayurveda Spa and Wellness Centres have emerged as sanctuaries where individuals seek solace and healing through the profound wisdom of Ayurvedic practices. This essay delves into the concept, offerings, and significance of Ayurveda Spa and Wellness Centres.

THE ESSENCE OF AYURVEDA SPA AND WELLNESS

Ayurveda Spa and Wellness Centres are places of rejuvenation and healing that blend traditional Ayurvedic principles with modern amenities. At their core, these centers aim to restore and maintain harmony within the individual. They recognize that well-being is not merely the absence of disease but a balanced state of physical, mental, and emotional health. Here's a closer look at what these centers offer:

Ayurvedic Therapies: The heart of Ayurveda Spa and Wellness Centres lies in the therapeutic treatments derived from ancient Ayurvedic texts. These treatments, which include Abhyanga (oil massage), Shirodhara (oil pouring on the forehead), and

Panchakarma (detoxification), are tailored to individual doshas (biological energies) to restore equilibrium.

Mind-Body Connection: Ayurveda places a strong emphasis on the mind-body connection. These centers often provide yoga and meditation classes to promote mental and emotional well-being. Guests can learn techniques to manage stress, enhance focus, and cultivate a tranquil mind.

Nutrition: Proper nutrition is a fundamental aspect of Ayurveda. Guests are guided in understanding their unique dietary needs based on their dosha, and wholesome Ayurvedic meals are served to nourish and balance the body.

Holistic Healing: Beyond physical health, Ayurveda Spa and Wellness Centres focus on overall wellness. They offer lifestyle counseling, personalized wellness plans, and herbal remedies to address various health concerns and maintain a balanced life.

Significance of Ayurveda Spa and Wellness Centres

The significance of Ayurveda Spa and Wellness Centres extends far beyond relaxation and rejuvenation. They serve as essential bridges between ancient wisdom and modern health needs:

Holistic Approach: Ayurveda takes a holistic approach to health, which aligns with the growing interest in holistic medicine and preventive healthcare worldwide. These centers offer an alternative to conventional medical practices by addressing the root causes of health issues.

Cultural Preservation: Ayurveda Spa and Wellness Centres contribute to the preservation of traditional knowledge and culture. They encourage the use of herbal remedies, Ayurvedic principles, and yoga, keeping these ancient practices alive and relevant.

Stress Management: In today's fast-paced world, stress and its associated health problems are prevalent. These centers offer effective stress management techniques, helping individuals cope with the demands of modern life.

Personalized Care: Ayurveda recognizes that each person is unique, and wellness should be tailored to individual needs. These centers provide personalized care, focusing on the individual's specific constitution and health goals.

Conclusion: Ayurveda Spa and Wellness Centres represent a harmonious blend of ancient wisdom and contemporary needs. They offer a refuge for individuals seeking holistic health, healing, and rejuvenation. In a world increasingly aware of the importance of well-being, these centers play a pivotal role in promoting health, balance, and spiritual nourishment, echoing the timeless wisdom of Ayurveda, the science of life.

ONLINE AYURVEDIC CONSULTATION

In recent years, the healthcare landscape has undergone a significant transformation with the advent of online platforms. Among the many changes, one that stands out is the rise of online Ayurvedic consultation. Ayurveda, an ancient holistic system of medicine originating in India, has found a new avenue for reaching people in need of its healing wisdom through digital means. This essay explores the evolution, benefits, challenges, and ethical considerations of online Ayurvedic consultation.

THE EVOLUTION OF ONLINE AYURVEDIC CONSULTATION

Traditionally, Ayurvedic medicine involved in-person consultations with experienced practitioners who would diagnose and provide treatment based on the principles of Ayurveda. However, with the growth of the internet and digital technology, Ayurvedic consultations have moved to online platforms. This transition has allowed individuals from around the world to access the expertise of Ayurvedic practitioners without geographical limitations.

BENEFITS OF ONLINE AYURVEDIC CONSULTATION

Accessibility: Online consultations break down geographical barriers, making Ayurvedic expertise available to individuals who may not have access to traditional Ayurvedic practitioners in their local area.

Convenience: Patients can schedule consultations at their convenience, eliminating the need to travel to a clinic. This convenience is particularly beneficial for individuals with busy schedules.

Privacy: Online consultations offer a degree of privacy that some patients may prefer when discussing personal health concerns.

Information Sharing: Digital platforms enable patients to share health records and information easily, which can aid in more accurate diagnoses and treatment plans.

CHALLENGES OF ONLINE AYURVEDIC CONSULTATION

Lack of Physical Examination: One of the primary challenges is the absence of a physical examination, which is crucial in Ayurvedic diagnosis. Practitioners may rely solely on verbal descriptions and images, which may not provide a comprehensive understanding of the patient's condition.

Misdiagnosis: Without the ability to physically examine patients, there is a risk of misdiagnosis, leading to inappropriate treatments.

Limited Herb Dispensation: Traditional Ayurvedic medicines often involve personalized herbal preparations. Online consultations may limit the practitioner's ability to create custom remedies.

ETHICAL CONSIDERATIONS

Informed Consent: Practitioners must ensure that patients fully understand the limitations of online consultations and the potential risks involved.

Privacy and Data Security: Online platforms should adhere to stringent privacy and data security measures to protect patient information.

Licensing and Regulation: Online Ayurvedic practitioners must adhere to the relevant legal and ethical guidelines, ensuring they are properly qualified and licensed to provide medical advice.

*****

Chapter 5

Ayurveda Manufacturing Units

योगादपिविषंतीक्ष्णमुत्तमं भेषजं भवेत्।
भेषजं चापि दुर्युक्तं तीक्ष्णं सम्पद्यते विषम्॥१२६॥

Yogaadapi visham tikshmuttam bheshajam bhavet, bheshjam chaapi duryuktam tiksham sampadhyate visham

Even an acute poison can become an excellent drug if it is properly administered. On the other hand, even a drug, if not properly administered, becomes an acute poison.

Charaka Sutra Sthana,Chapter 24, verse 126

HIGHLIGHTS

The manufacturing of classical Ayurvedic formulations blends ancient wisdom with modern standards to produce safe and effective remedies for holistic well-being.

The manufacturing of proprietary Ayurvedic formulations, Veterinary and Poultry Medicines, Herbal Extracts, Ayurvedic FMCG Products, Skin and Beauty Products, Herbal Supplements and Nutraceuricals, offers a unique opportunity to meet the growing global demand for natural and holistic healthcare products, leveraging traditional trust, lower regulatory hurdles, cost-effective production, export potential, and alignment with the health and wellness trend.

MANUFACTURING OF AYURVEDIC MEDICINES

The manufacturing of Ayurvedic medicines is a meticulous process that combines ancient knowledge with modern standards to produce safe and effective herbal remedies. In this essay, we will explore the key steps and considerations involved in the manufacturing of Ayurvedic medicines.

Selection of Herbs: Ayurvedic medicines are primarily plant-based, and the selection of herbs is a crucial step. Experienced Ayurvedic practitioners and manufacturers choose herbs based on their therapeutic properties and compatibility with the patient's constitution (Prakriti).

Sourcing of Raw Materials: High-quality raw materials are essential for effective medicines. Manufacturers must ensure that herbs and other ingredients are sourced from reputable suppliers who adhere to quality and safety standards.

Cleaning and Processing: Raw herbs are often cleaned and processed to remove impurities, such as dust and foreign matter. This step ensures the purity of the ingredients.

Herbal Formulations: Ayurvedic medicines are often a combination of several herbs and minerals. The specific formulation and proportion of ingredients are carefully determined, often following ancient Ayurvedic texts.

Extraction Methods: Various extraction methods are used to obtain the active constituents from herbs. Techniques like boiling, fermentation, and drying are employed to extract and concentrate the medicinal properties.

Standardization and Quality Control: Ayurvedic medicines must meet quality standards for consistency and efficacy. This involves testing for purity, potency, and absence of contaminants.

Manufacturing Process: The actual manufacturing process may include making pastes, powders, tablets, or oils. Care is taken to maintain aseptic conditions and ensure that the medicines are produced under strict hygiene standards.

Preservation and Packaging: To maintain the shelf life of Ayurvedic medicines, natural preservatives and packaging that protect the products from environmental factors are used. Traditional methods often involve storing medicines in glass containers or clay pots.

Regulatory Compliance: In many countries, Ayurvedic medicines are subject to regulatory oversight to ensure they meet safety and quality standards. Compliance with relevant regulations is essential for market approval.

Research and Development: Ongoing research is conducted to enhance Ayurvedic formulations, validate their efficacy, and adapt them to modern healthcare needs.

Traditional Knowledge Preservation: Ayurvedic manufacturers often work in collaboration with Ayurvedic experts to preserve and pass on the traditional knowledge related to herbal remedies.

Sustainability: Sustainable practices in herb cultivation and harvesting are crucial to ensure a consistent supply of raw materials without depleting natural resources.

Manufacturing Ayurvedic medicines is a delicate blend of ancient wisdom and modern science. It requires a deep understanding of Ayurvedic principles, strict adherence to quality control measures, and compliance with regulatory standards. Ayurveda continues to gain recognition globally for its holistic approach to health, and the manufacturing of Ayurvedic medicines plays a pivotal role in making these remedies accessible to those seeking natural and traditional healthcare solutions.

MANUFACTURING OF AYURVEDIC FMCG AND BEAUTY PRODUCTS

The manufacturing of Ayurvedic Fast-Moving Consumer Goods (FMCG) and beauty products is a complex process that combines traditional herbal knowledge with modern manufacturing techniques to create products that cater to the growing demand for natural and holistic wellness. This essay will delve into the key aspects of the manufacturing process for Ayurvedic FMCG and beauty products, highlighting the unique blend of tradition and innovation that characterizes this industry.

1. **Ingredient Sourcing and Selection:** The foundation of Ayurvedic product manufacturing lies in the careful selection of natural ingredients. Ayurveda, an ancient Indian system of medicine, emphasizes the use of herbs, minerals, and other organic substances. Manufacturers source ingredients from various regions, ensuring their authenticity and quality. These ingredients are chosen based on their therapeutic properties, which align with the principles of Ayurveda.

2. **Traditional Knowledge Integration:** Manufacturers often collaborate with Ayurvedic experts and traditional practitioners to ensure the efficacy of their products.

These experts provide insights into the traditional healing properties of ingredients and the synergies between them. This integration of ancient wisdom is essential to maintaining the authenticity of Ayurvedic products.

3. **Manufacturing Facilities:** State-of-the-art manufacturing facilities are crucial for maintaining quality and consistency. These facilities must adhere to Good Manufacturing Practices (GMP) and other industry standards. The processes are designed to minimize contamination and ensure product purity.

4. **Formulation Development:** Ayurvedic formulations are developed through a combination of modern scientific research and traditional Ayurvedic texts. Formulation scientists work to optimize the combination of ingredients, proportions, and preparation methods to maximize the product's effectiveness.

5. **Quality Control:** Rigorous quality control measures are implemented at various stages of manufacturing. This includes testing for the presence of heavy metals, microbes, and other contaminants. Additionally, the products are assessed for stability, shelf-life, and effectiveness.

6. **Regulatory Compliance:** Manufacturers must comply with regulatory requirements specific to Ayurvedic products. This may involve adhering to guidelines from health authorities, such as the Food and Drug Administration (FDA) in various countries. Compliance ensures product safety and legality.

7. **Packaging and Labeling:** The packaging of Ayurvedic FMCG and beauty products is designed to protect the product from environmental factors and preserve its potency. Labels

include comprehensive information about the product's ingredients, usage instructions, and any certifications it may have, such as organic or cruelty-free.

8. **Sustainability and Ethical Practices:** Many manufacturers prioritize sustainable and ethical practices, such as sourcing ingredients responsibly, reducing waste, and supporting local communities. These practices align with the eco-conscious values of many consumers.

9. **Market Adaptation:** Manufacturers keep an eye on market trends and consumer preferences to introduce new products or reformulate existing ones. This ensures that Ayurvedic FMCG and beauty products remain competitive in a dynamic market.

10. **Research and Development:** Ongoing research and development efforts are crucial to improving existing products and developing innovative solutions. Manufacturers invest in scientific studies to validate the therapeutic benefits of Ayurvedic ingredients.

In conclusion, the manufacturing of Ayurvedic FMCG and beauty products is a delicate balance of tradition and modernity. It combines the wisdom of Ayurveda with advanced manufacturing techniques and quality control standards to produce holistic wellness and beauty solutions. This industry reflects a growing global interest in natural, sustainable, and culturally rich approaches to self-care and well-being.

MANUFACTURING OF HERBAL EXTRACTS, SUPPLEMENTS AND NUTRACEUTICALS

The manufacturing of herbal extracts, supplements, and nutraceuticals plays a crucial role in the healthcare and wellness industry. These products have gained popularity due to their perceived natural and holistic benefits. This essay will explore the processes involved in manufacturing these items and highlight their significance in promoting health and well-being.

Herbal extracts, supplements, and nutraceuticals are typically derived from various plant sources, including herbs, fruits, and vegetables. The manufacturing process can be broken down into several key steps:

Sourcing and Selection of Raw Materials: The first step involves carefully selecting and sourcing the plant materials. Quality is essential, as it directly affects the final product's efficacy. Cultivation, harvesting, and post-harvest handling must meet stringent standards to ensure the highest quality.

Extraction: Once the raw materials are obtained, the active compounds need to be extracted. This can be done through various methods such as maceration, percolation, or supercritical fluid extraction. The choice of extraction method depends on the specific plant and desired compounds.

Standardization: To ensure consistency and potency, the extracted substances are often standardized to contain a particular concentration of active ingredients. This step is critical in achieving the desired therapeutic effects.

Formulation: The extracted substances are then formulated into various product forms, such as capsules, tablets, tinctures, or powders. Formulation may involve combining multiple extracts or adding excipients to create a stable, easy-to-use product.

Quality Control and Testing: Stringent quality control measures are implemented throughout the manufacturing process. This includes testing for purity, potency, and the absence of contaminants such as heavy metals, pesticides, and microbial organisms.

Packaging and Labeling: The final products are packaged in a way that preserves their integrity and potency. Labeling is crucial to provide consumers with information on proper usage, dosage, and potential contraindications.

Manufacturing herbal extracts, supplements, and nutraceuticals serves a vital role in promoting health and wellness. These products offer a range of benefits:

Holistic Health Approach: Herbal extracts and nutraceuticals are often perceived as a more natural and holistic approach to health, addressing both prevention and treatment of various health conditions.

Nutrient Supplementation: They can provide essential vitamins, minerals, and phytonutrients that may be lacking in an individual's diet, helping to maintain overall health and well-being.

Reduced Side Effects: Many herbal supplements have fewer side effects compared to synthetic pharmaceuticals, making them an attractive option for those seeking alternatives to traditional medications.

Preventive Health Measures: Nutraceuticals can play a role in preventive health by providing antioxidants and compounds that may reduce the risk of chronic diseases.

However, it's essential to note that the manufacturing of herbal extracts, supplements, and nutraceuticals is subject to regulation and quality control to ensure product safety and effectiveness. Manufacturers should adhere to Good Manufacturing Practices (GMP) and meet industry standards.

In conclusion, the manufacturing of herbal extracts, supplements, and nutraceuticals is a critical aspect of the healthcare industry. These products offer a natural and holistic approach to health and well-being, providing a wide range of benefits while requiring strict adherence to quality control and regulatory standards to ensure consumer safety and product efficacy.

MANUFACTURING OF AYURVEDIC VETERINARY AND POULTRY MEDICINES

The manufacturing of Ayurvedic veterinary and poultry medicines can be a lucrative business if approached strategically. Here are some factors to consider:

Market Demand: Assess the demand for Ayurvedic veterinary and poultry medicines in your target market. Conduct market research to understand the needs of farmers and veterinary professionals.

Quality Control: Ensure that your products meet quality standards and regulations. Consistency in quality is essential to gain trust in this industry.

Research and Development: Invest in research to develop effective Ayurvedic formulations for animal health. Innovations can set you apart from competitors.

Regulatory Compliance: Familiarize yourself with the regulatory requirements for manufacturing and selling veterinary medicines in your region. Compliance is crucial to avoid legal issues.

Distribution Network: Establish a strong distribution network to reach your target customers effectively. Consider collaborating with veterinarians and poultry farmers.

Marketing and Branding: Build a strong brand image and market your products effectively. Highlight the benefits of Ayurvedic medicines, such as natural ingredients and minimal side effects.

Competitive Pricing: Price your products competitively while ensuring profitability. Consider the pricing strategies of your competitors.

Sustainability: Emphasize eco-friendly and sustainable practices in your manufacturing process to attract environmentally conscious customers.

Education and Training: Offer training and educational resources to veterinarians and poultry farmers about the benefits and proper usage of your products.

Adaptability: Stay updated with the latest trends and developments in Ayurvedic medicine and the veterinary industry to adapt and grow your business.

*****

Chapter 6

Ayurveda Tourism and Hospitality

द्विविधमेव खलु सर्वं सच्चासच्च; तस्य चतुर्विधा परीक्षा–
आप्तोपदेशः, प्रत्यक्षम्, अनुमानं, युक्तिश्चेति॥१७॥

Dwidhameva khalu sarvam sacchasachh, tasya chaturvidha pariksha – Aaptopdeshah, Pratyaksham, Anumanam, Yuktishcheti

All things of the universe can be divided into two.

Sat – true / existent

Asat – untrue / non-existent

These can be examined by means of –

Aptopadesha – scriptural testimony (words of enlightened, realized souls),

Pratyaksha – direct perception using the sense organs,

Anumana – inference, or guessing with reason,

Yukti – reasoning with intelligence.

Charaka Sutra Sthana, Chapter 11, verse 17

HIGHLIGHTS

Combining Ayurveda with tourism provides holistic wellness and cultural immersion.

Key elements include wellness retreats and eco-friendly practices, creating a unique and enriching experience for travelers.

SETTING UP AN WELLNESS RESORT

The wellness industry is experiencing rapid growth worldwide, and Ayurveda, the ancient Indian system of natural healing, has gained popularity as a holistic approach to health and well-being. Setting up an Ayurveda and Wellness Resort can be a rewarding venture, combining the principles of Ayurveda with luxurious accommodations and a serene environment to offer a unique experience for guests. In this essay, we will explore the steps and considerations involved in establishing such a business.

I. MARKET RESEARCH AND FEASIBILITY STUDY

The first step in establishing an Ayurveda and Wellness Resort is to conduct thorough market research and a feasibility study. This should involve analyzing the demand for wellness services, identifying your target market, and assessing the competition in the area. Understanding the market dynamics will help in crafting a business plan tailored to the needs of your potential customers.

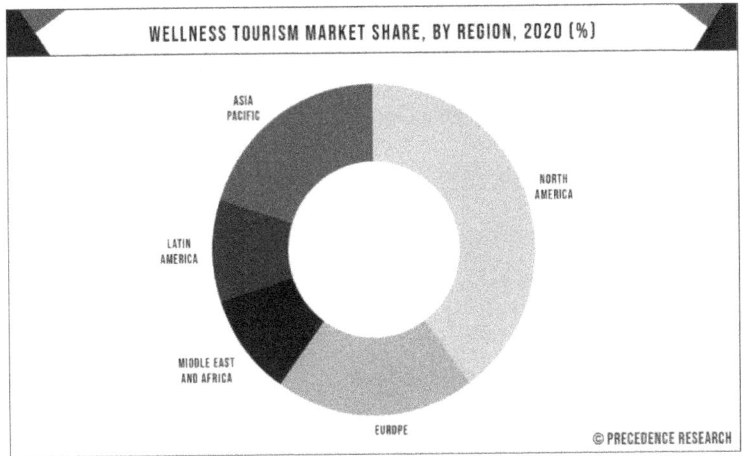

Fig: 6.1 Image showing wellness tourism market share by region

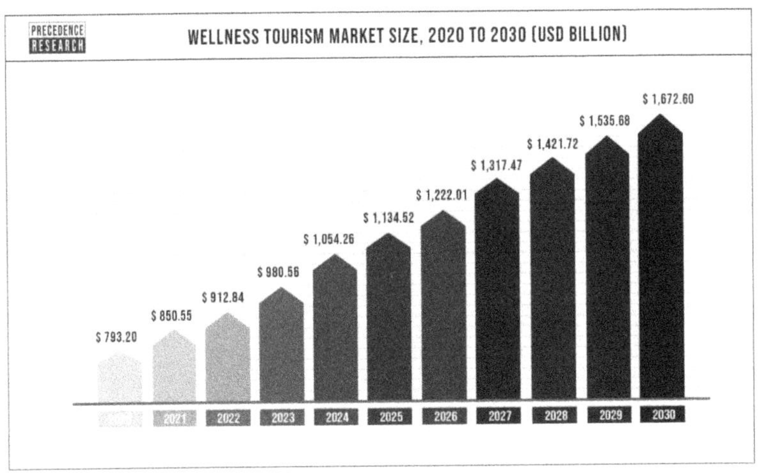

Fig: 6.2 Image showing wellness tourism market share by revenue

II. BUSINESS PLAN

Develop a comprehensive business plan that outlines your resort's vision, mission, and goals. Include a detailed description of your services, pricing strategy, and marketing plan. The plan should also address the legal and regulatory requirements for operating a wellness resort, such as permits, licenses, and compliance with health and safety standards.

III. LOCATION SELECTION

Choosing the right location is crucial for the success of your Ayurveda and Wellness Resort. The site should be in a peaceful and natural setting, away from the noise and pollution of urban areas. Access to clean water and a pollution-free environment is essential for providing authentic Ayurvedic treatments.

IV. INFRASTRUCTURE AND AMENITIES

Invest in well-designed and comfortable accommodations, treatment facilities, yoga and meditation spaces, and a restaurant serving healthy Ayurvedic cuisine. Ensure that the resort has well-trained staff, including Ayurvedic doctors, therapists, and yoga instructors. Consider eco-friendly practices and sustainable construction to appeal to environmentally conscious guests.

V. AYURVEDIC SERVICES

The core of your resort's offerings will be Ayurvedic services such as Panchakarma detoxification, Ayurvedic consultations, herbal treatments, and personalized wellness plans. You should also offer yoga, meditation, and other holistic therapies to promote overall well-being.

VI. MARKETING AND BRANDING

Develop a strong brand identity that reflects the essence of Ayurveda and wellness. Implement a digital marketing strategy, create a user-friendly website, and engage in social media marketing. Partner with travel agencies, wellness influencers, and local businesses to promote your resort.

VII. REGULATORY COMPLIANCE

Comply with all relevant regulations and obtain the necessary permits and licenses. This includes adhering to healthcare and safety standards and ensuring the qualifications of your Ayurvedic practitioners and therapists.

VIII. SUSTAINABILITY

Incorporate sustainable practices in your resort's operations, such as energy efficiency, waste reduction, and water conservation. Eco-friendly initiatives not only appeal to environmentally conscious guests but also help reduce operational costs in the long run.

IX. FINANCIAL MANAGEMENT

Implement robust financial management systems to monitor expenses, revenue, and profitability. Establish pricing strategies that reflect the value of your services while remaining competitive in the market. Consider financial projections and contingency plans to address unexpected challenges.

Conclusion: Setting up an Ayurveda and Wellness Resort as a business is a holistic and rewarding endeavor that can contribute to the well-being of your guests. With the right planning, location, services, and commitment to sustainability, your resort can become a haven for those seeking authentic Ayurvedic treatments and a rejuvenating wellness experience. Remember that success in this industry requires dedication, continuous learning, and a genuine passion for promoting health and happiness.

BLENDING TOURISM AND TRADITIONAL AYURVEDA TREATMENT

Blending tourism and traditional Ayurveda treatment can provide a unique and holistic experience for travelers. Tourists seeking wellness and cultural immersion can explore the following ideas:

Cultural Immersion: Offer opportunities for tourists to engage in local customs and traditions, such as participating in traditional Ayurvedic rituals and learning about herbal medicines.

Ayurvedic Tourism Packages: Create packages that combine guided tours of cultural sites with Ayurvedic treatments, allowing tourists to enjoy the best of both worlds.

Eco-Friendly Practices: Promote eco-friendly practices and sustainable tourism to align with Ayurveda's holistic principles and respect for nature.

Ayurvedic Workshops: Offer workshops where tourists can learn about Ayurvedic principles, herbal remedies, and even prepare Ayurvedic dishes.

Customized Experiences: Tailor treatments and activities to tourists' individual needs and preferences, enhancing their overall well-being.

By combining traditional Ayurveda with tourism, you can create a compelling and enriching experience that appeals to health-conscious travelers while preserving and sharing the rich heritage of Ayurvedic practices.

*****

Chapter 7

Trading In Ayurveda

इह खलु पुरुषेणानुपहतसत्त्वबुद्धिपौरुषपराक्रमेण हितमिह
चामुष्मिंश्च लोके समनुपश्यता तिस्र एषणाः पर्येष्टव्या भवन्ति|

तद्यथा– प्राणैषणा, धनैषणा, परलोकैषणेति||३||

Eh khalu
purushenanupahatsatvabudhipaurushparakramen hitmih
chamushmimshcha loke samnupashyata tisra aiyeshnah
paryeshtavya bhavanti

Tadhyata- pranyeshna, dhanyeshna, parlokyeshnayti

The 3 basic pursuits of life

A person of normal mental faculty, intelligence, strength, and energy, has to seek three basic desires of life….

Praneshana – the desire to live,

Dhaneshana – the desire to earn,

Paralokeshana – the desire to have a superior position after death

Charaka Sutra Sthana, Chapter 11, verse 3

HIGHLIGHTS

Retailing wholesaling and export of Ayurvedic medicines are pivotal in popularizing Ayurvedic remedies and wellness products, contributing to the domestic and global growth of this traditional system of medicine.

To succeed in the online Ayurveda e-commerce business, prioritize market research, quality products, compliance, and effective online presence to build customer trust and promote health and well-being.

RETAIL AND WHOLESALE AYURVEDA STORES

Retail and wholesale Ayurveda stores play a pivotal role in making these traditional remedies and wellness products accessible to a wider audience. This essay explores the significance, evolution, and impact of such stores in promoting Ayurveda.

THE GROWTH OF AYURVEDA STORES

In recent years, there has been a surge in the demand for Ayurvedic products and treatments globally. This has led to the emergence of numerous retail and wholesale Ayurveda stores. These stores offer a wide array of Ayurvedic products, including herbal remedies, dietary supplements, skincare and haircare products, and various holistic wellness items. Their popularity can be attributed to several factors:

Increasing Awareness: People are becoming more health-conscious and are seeking alternatives to conventional medicine.

Ayurveda's focus on natural and holistic healing resonates with this trend.

Safety and Efficacy: Ayurvedic remedies are often considered safe and effective with minimal side effects when used correctly. This reputation boosts their demand.

Globalization: The globalization of Ayurveda has expanded its reach. Ayurvedic products are now available worldwide, thanks to these stores.

Wellness Trend: The modern emphasis on holistic wellness has led to the incorporation of Ayurvedic practices, such as yoga and meditation, into daily routines. Ayurveda stores complement this trend by offering related products and services.

RETAIL AYURVEDA STORES

Retail Ayurveda stores cater to individual consumers, offering a wide range of Ayurvedic products. These stores often have knowledgeable staff who can provide guidance and recommendations based on the customer's specific needs and constitution. Products include herbal supplements, oils, teas, cosmetics, and more. Some Ayurveda stores also provide consultation services with Ayurvedic practitioners.

WHOLESALE AYURVEDA STORES

Wholesale Ayurveda stores serve a different purpose. They supply Ayurvedic products in bulk to various retail outlets, wellness centers, spas, and even healthcare facilities. These wholesalers often work directly with Ayurvedic manufacturers and distributors. Their role is critical in ensuring that Ayurvedic products are readily available in various markets.

IMPACT AND CHALLENGES

The impact of retail and wholesale Ayurveda stores is significant in promoting traditional wellness. They have made Ayurvedic products accessible to a global audience, thereby contributing to the growth of Ayurveda as a global industry. These stores also help preserve and promote the knowledge and practices of this ancient system of medicine.

However, there are challenges to address. Quality control and standardization of Ayurvedic products are crucial to maintain the safety and efficacy of these remedies. Additionally, the need for proper regulation to prevent misleading claims and ensure product authenticity is an ongoing concern.

Conclusion: Retail and wholesale Ayurveda stores play a pivotal role in the resurgence of Ayurveda in the modern world. They make traditional remedies and holistic wellness products accessible to a global audience. While they have brought numerous benefits, there is a responsibility to maintain quality, authenticity, and ethical marketing practices within the Ayurveda industry. As long as these challenges are met, Ayurveda will continue to thrive as a holistic approach to health and wellness.

ONLINE AYURVEDA E-COMMERCE STORES

Starting an online Ayurveda e-commerce store can be a viable business idea. Here are some key points to consider:

Market Research: Understand the demand for Ayurvedic products in your target market. Research competitors and identify your unique selling proposition.

Product Selection: Carefully select a range of Ayurvedic products to sell, including herbal supplements, skincare, haircare, and wellness products. Ensure they meet safety and quality standards.

Regulations and Compliance: Comply with local regulations regarding the sale of herbal and Ayurvedic products. Ensure that your products are properly tested and labeled.

Supplier Relationships: Establish relationships with reputable suppliers or consider manufacturing your own products. Quality is crucial in the Ayurvedic market.

E-commerce Platform: Choose a reliable e-commerce platform to set up your online store. Ensure it's user-friendly and mobile-responsive.

Website Design: Invest in professional website design for an attractive and user-friendly online store. Make it easy for customers to navigate and make purchases.

Payment Processing: Set up secure and convenient payment processing options for customers.

Content and Education: Provide informative content on your website about Ayurveda, the benefits of specific products, and how to use them. This can help build trust and loyalty.

Marketing: Develop a marketing strategy that includes SEO, social media, email marketing, and possibly influencer partnerships to reach your target audience.

Customer Service: Offer excellent customer service, including quick response to inquiries and addressing customer concerns.

Shipping and Fulfillment: Plan how you will handle shipping and order fulfillment. Offer reasonable shipping rates and delivery times.

Customer Reviews and Feedback: Encourage customers to leave reviews and provide feedback. Positive reviews can boost your credibility.

Data Security: Ensure the security of customer data and payment information.

Scaling: As your business grows, be prepared to scale up your operations and potentially expand your product offerings.

Legal Considerations: Consult with legal experts to understand any specific regulations for selling herbal and Ayurvedic products in your region.

Remember that the success of your Ayurveda e-commerce store will depend on the quality of your products, your marketing efforts, and the trust you build with your customers. It's essential to operate ethically and provide products that genuinely benefit your customers' health and well-being.

EXPORT OF AYURVEDIC HERBS AND MEDICINES

The global Ayurvedic herbs market size was valued at $9.5 billion in 2020 and is anticipated to reach $21.6 billion by 2028, with a CAGR of 10.8% during the forecast period. Ayurvedic herbs are elements of the Ayurveda, also called as traditional practice of medicine. Ayurvedic herbs are an important component of the traditional Indian system of medicine. They're thought to protect the body from disease and offer a variety of health benefits, including improved digestion and mental health, diabetes, infectious diseases, and cardiovascular diseases, among others.

Exporting Ayurvedic herbs and medicines can be a viable business opportunity. Here are some key steps to consider:

Research and Compliance: Understand the regulations and compliance requirements for exporting Ayurvedic products. Ensure that your products meet quality standards and are compliant with international regulations.

Quality Sourcing: Source herbs and ingredients from reliable and certified suppliers. Quality is crucial in the Ayurvedic industry.

Manufacturing Facilities: Establish or partner with manufacturing facilities that adhere to good manufacturing practices (GMP) for Ayurvedic medicines.

Documentation: Prepare all necessary documentation, including product certificates, safety data, and compliance records for export.

Market Research: Identify target markets. Research the demand for Ayurvedic products in those markets and the competition.

Distribution Channels: Decide on your distribution strategy, whether you'll sell directly to retailers, distributors, or online.

Build Relationships: Cultivate relationships with international distributors, importers, and regulatory bodies to facilitate exports.

Branding and Packaging: Invest in professional branding and packaging. Ayurvedic products are often perceived as premium, so presentation matters.

Certifications: Consider obtaining relevant certifications like Organic, Halal, or Kosher to expand your market reach.

Logistics and Shipping: Plan your logistics for international shipping, including choosing reliable freight and shipping companies.

Market Entry Strategy: Decide whether you'll start with a particular product range or focus on a specific geographic region.

Promotion and Marketing: Invest in marketing and promotion tailored to your target markets, highlighting the benefits of Ayurvedic products.

Compliance with Trademarks and Patents: Ensure your products do not infringe on trademarks or patents in the target markets.

Financial Planning: Develop a robust financial plan that includes budgeting for marketing, shipping, and regulatory compliance.

Risk Assessment: Assess the potential risks and challenges in the export business, such as currency fluctuations, changing regulations, and cultural differences.

Adaptability: Be prepared to adapt to the preferences and regulations of different countries.

Continuous Learning: Stay updated with the latest developments in Ayurveda and the global herbal medicine market.

Remember that success in the Ayurvedic export business requires a deep understanding of the science and traditional practices of Ayurveda, a commitment to quality, and compliance with international standards and regulations.

*****

Chapter 8

Herbs Agriculture and Farming

त्रय उपस्तम्भा इति-आहारः, स्वप्नो, ब्रह्मचर्यमिति; एभिस्त्रिभिर्युक्तियुक्तैरुपस्तब्धमुपस्तम्भैः शरीरं

बलवर्णोपचयोपचितमनुवर्ततेयावदायुःसंस्कारात् संस्कारमहितमनुपसेवमानस्य, य इहैवोपदेक्ष्यते॥३५॥

Triya Upstambha iti- Aaharah,
swapno, brahmacharyamiti,
aibhistribhiryuktiyuktairupstabdhamupastambhayai
shariram balvarnopchayopachitamnuvartateyaavadayu
sanskaraat samskaramhitanupsevamanasya ya
ihaivopdekshyate

The three supports of life are the following.

Ahara – food

Nidra – sleep

Brahmacharya – moderation of sexual intercourse (neither very frequently nor infrequent)

Healthy habits pertaining to food, sleep, and celibacy leads to good complexion, growth and full health for the full span of one's life.

Charaka Sutra Sthana, Chapter 11, verse 35

HIGHLIGHTS

Key steps for success in cultivating and selling organic herbs and plants include market research, organic certification, sustainable cultivation, and effective marketing.

Profitability in this business is influenced by factors like herb selection, local demand, and cost management, making thorough market research and financial planning crucial.

GLOBAL FRESH HERBS MARKET OVERVIEW

The Fresh Herbs Market Size was valued at USD 142.1 Billion in 2022. The Fresh Herbs market industry is projected to grow from USD 165.2 Billion in 2023 to USD 407.9 Billion by 2032, exhibiting a compound annual growth rate (CAGR) of 16.26% during the forecast period (2023 - 2032). Increased awareness about the health benefits of fresh herbs and rising preference for packaged fresh herbs are the key market drivers enhancing the growth of market.

CULTIVATING AND SELLING ORGANIC HERBS AND PLANTS

Herbs and plants can be a profitable niche, especially if you focus on high-demand varieties, such as culinary herbs, medicinal plants, or unique ornamental species. Organic herbs often command premium prices due to their perceived quality and health benefits.

Market Research: Identify your target market and understand what herbs and plants are in demand. Consider both culinary and medicinal herbs, as well as decorative plants.

Location: Choose a suitable location for cultivation, whether it's a backyard garden, greenhouse, or a larger farm. Ensure it meets the organic certification requirements if applicable.

Organic Certification: If you want to sell organic herbs, consider getting organic certification. This can boost your credibility with eco-conscious consumers.

Cultivation: Learn about the specific requirements for each herb or plant you plan to grow, including soil, water, and sunlight needs. Implement sustainable and organic farming practices.

Seed and Plant Selection: Carefully select high-quality seeds or seedlings to ensure healthy and robust growth.

Pest and Disease Management: Develop organic pest and disease management strategies to avoid the use of synthetic chemicals.

Harvesting: Time your harvests carefully to ensure the highest quality and potency of your herbs and plants.

Packaging: Invest in attractive and eco-friendly packaging to appeal to customers.

Marketing: Create a brand, develop an online presence, and market your products through farmers' markets, local stores, or online platforms.

Compliance: Understand and comply with local regulations and permits related to agriculture and sales.

Sustainability: Emphasize your commitment to sustainability and eco-friendliness, as it can be a selling point for organic products.

Customer Engagement: Build relationships with your customers and seek feedback to improve your products and services.

The profitability of cultivating and selling organic herbs and plants can vary widely depending on several factors, including the types of herbs and plants you choose to grow, the market demand in your region, your marketing and distribution strategies, and your ability to manage costs effective Plant.

Success in this business also depends on your ability to scale production, control expenses, and build a strong customer base. It's important to conduct thorough market research and financial planning to assess the potential profitability in your specific area.

PROFITABLE HERBS AND CULTIVATION

Herbs have been an integral part of human civilization for centuries. Beyond their culinary and medicinal uses, herbs can be a profitable venture for those interested in cultivating them. In this essay, we will explore the names of some of the most profitable herbs and delve into the cultivation process, shedding light on the steps to a successful herb farming business.

PROFITABLE HERB NAMES

Lavender (Lavandula angustifolia): Lavender is a versatile herb with a wide range of applications, from essential oils to cosmetics. It thrives in well-drained, sandy soil and requires full sun exposure.

Ginseng (Panax ginseng): Ginseng, known for its medicinal properties, is a high-value herb. It typically grows in the shaded, wooded areas of North America and Asia, requiring specific soil conditions.

Saffron (Crocus sativus): Saffron, one of the most expensive spices globally, comes from the flower's stigma. It can be cultivated in well-drained, loamy soil in areas with mild winters.

Oregano (Origanum vulgare): Oregano is a popular culinary herb with a robust market. It prefers well-drained, sandy soil and full sun.

Mint (Mentha spp.): Mint, used for teas and culinary purposes, is a hardy herb that can grow in various soil types but thrives in rich, moist soil.

Rosemary (Rosmarinus officinalis): Rosemary is a popular culinary herb with a robust flavor. It's drought-tolerant and thrives in well-drained soil with full sun exposure.

Chives (Allium schoenoprasum): Chives are used in cooking and have a mild onion flavor. They can be grown in a variety of soil types and prefer partial shade.

Stevia (Stevia rebaudiana): Stevia is a natural sweetener, and there's a growing demand for it in the health-conscious market. It requires well-drained, loamy soil and warm conditions.

Coriander (Coriandrum sativum): Coriander, both its leaves (cilantro) and seeds, is a common culinary herb. It grows best in well-drained soil with partial shade in hot climates.

Echinacea (Echinacea purpurea): Echinacea is known for its potential health benefits. It thrives in well-drained soil and requires full sun.

Lemongrass (Cymbopogon citratus): Lemongrass is used in cooking and for its aromatic properties. It prefers well-drained, sandy soil and full sun.

Valerian (Valeriana officinalis): Valerian is known for its calming properties and is used in herbal remedies. It grows well in moist, fertile soil in partially shaded areas.

Thyme (Thymus vulgaris): Thyme is a versatile herb used in cooking and aromatherapy. It prefers well-drained, slightly alkaline soil and full sun.

Turmeric (Curcuma longa): Turmeric is sought after for its health benefits and vibrant color. It grows best in well-drained, loamy soil in tropical or subtropical regions.

Catnip (Nepeta cataria): Catnip is not just for feline friends; it's also used in herbal teas. It grows well in various soil types and full sun.

Lemongrass (Cymbopogon citratus): Lemongrass is used in culinary dishes and for its aromatic properties. It thrives in well-drained, sandy soil and requires full sun.

Aloe Vera (Aloe barbadensis miller): Aloe Vera is known for its healing properties and is used in skincare products. It prefers well-drained, sandy soil and lots of sunlight.

Chamomile (Matricaria chamomilla): Chamomile is used for making herbal teas and is valued for its calming effects. It grows best in well-drained soil with partial sun.

Lemon Balm (Melissa officinalis): Lemon Balm is a lemon-scented herb often used in teas and for aromatherapy. It prefers well-drained soil and partial shade.

Tarragon (Artemisia dracunculus): Tarragon is a popular culinary herb with a unique anise-like flavor. It grows well in well-drained, slightly alkaline soil with full sun.

Marshmallow (Althaea officinalis): Marshmallow is known for its soothing properties and is used in herbal remedies. It thrives in moist, rich soil and partial sun.

Each of these herbs has unique requirements and characteristics. Consider the local climate and market demand when choosing which herbs to cultivate. Proper care and attention to their specific growing conditions can make herb farming a profitable endeavor.

CULTIVATION PROCESS

Site Selection: Choose a suitable location with the right soil type and exposure to sunlight. Conduct a soil test to ensure it meets the herb's requirements.

Seed Selection: Purchase high-quality seeds or plant cuttings from reputable sources. Ensure they are disease-free.

Soil Preparation: Prepare the soil by removing weeds and rocks. Depending on the herb, amend the soil with organic matter, sand, or other materials to improve drainage or fertility.

Planting: Follow specific guidelines for each herb's planting depth and spacing. Water thoroughly after planting to establish the roots.

Watering: Herbs have varying water needs. Some, like lavender, prefer drier conditions, while others, like mint, require regular watering. Adapt your watering schedule accordingly.

Fertilization: Use organic or specific herb fertilizers to promote healthy growth. Be cautious not to over-fertilize, as it can negatively impact the herbs.

Pest and Disease Management: Regularly inspect the herbs for pests and diseases. Use organic or chemical treatments as necessary to protect your crop.

Harvesting: Harvest herbs at the right time to maximize their flavor and potency. This timing varies for each herb. For example, basil is best harvested before it flowers, while ginseng takes several years to mature.

Drying and Processing: After harvesting, properly dry and process the herbs to maintain their quality. For saffron, delicate handling during the harvesting and drying process is crucial.

Marketing and Sales: Develop a marketing strategy to sell your herbs. Consider selling them fresh, dried, or processed into value-added products like essential oils or spice blends. Establish a network with local markets, restaurants, or online platforms.

Conclusion: Cultivating profitable herbs requires careful planning, attention to detail, and knowledge of specific growing conditions for each herb. By selecting the right herb varieties and following best cultivation practices, individuals can turn herb farming into a profitable and rewarding venture. The diversity of herbs and their applications in various industries make this agricultural pursuit a promising option for those looking to enter the world of herb cultivation.

*****

Chapter 9

Research and Innovation In Ayurveda

विकारो धातुवैषम्यं, साम्यं प्रकृतिरुच्यते।
सुखसञ्ज्ञकमारोग्यं, विकारो दुःखमेव च॥४॥

Vikarodhatuvaishamayam, samyam prakritiruchyate,
sukhsangyakamarogyam, vikarodukhmev cha

Definition of health and disease:

Any disturbance in the equilibrium of Dhatus (Tridosha, body tissues and waste products) is known as disease.

The state of their equilibrium is health. Happiness indicates health and pain indicates disease.

Charaka Sutra Sthana,Chapter 9, verse 4

HIGHLIGHTS

Innovative product and treatment methodology development involves rigorous steps including market research, IP protection, team building, funding, compliance, testing, marketing, collaborations, scalability, and continuous innovation for success in sectors like healthcare and technology.

Developing equipment and software for Ayurvedic diagnosis and treatment involves extensive research, collaboration with experts, regulatory compliance, and ongoing improvement while respecting traditional principles and practices.

DEVELOP INNOVATIVE PRODUCTS AND TREATMENT METHODOLOGY

Developing innovative products and treatment methodologies as a business can be a promising venture, especially in sectors like healthcare, biotechnology, or technology. Here are some key steps to consider:

Market Research: Understand the needs and demands in your target market. Identify gaps or problems that your products or methodologies can address.

Intellectual Property: Protect your innovations through patents, trademarks, or copyrights to secure your competitive advantage.

Team Building: Assemble a team with diverse expertise in research, development, and business operations.

Funding: Seek funding from investors, grants, or venture capital to support research and development.

Regulatory Compliance: Be aware of and comply with regulatory requirements, especially in healthcare and biotechnology.

Prototyping and Testing: Develop prototypes and conduct rigorous testing to ensure safety and effectiveness.

Marketing and Branding: Create a strong brand and marketing strategy to build awareness and trust in your products or methodologies.

Collaborations: Partner with research institutions, healthcare providers, or other industry players for validation and distribution.

Scalability: Plan for scalability to meet growing demand as your business succeeds.

Continuous Innovation: Stay updated with the latest research and industry trends to adapt and improve your offerings.

Remember, the development of innovative products and treatment methodologies often involves significant research and development, regulatory hurdles, and market challenges. However, successful ventures can have a positive impact on society and generate substantial revenue.

DEVELOP NEW EQUIPMENT AND SOFTWARE FOR DIAGNOSIS AND TREATMENT

Creating new equipment and software for diagnosis and treatment in the field of Ayurveda can be a valuable venture. Here are some steps to consider:

Research and Development: Start by conducting in-depth research into Ayurvedic principles, diagnosis, and treatment methods. Understand the specific needs and challenges in Ayurvedic healthcare.

Collaborate with Ayurvedic Experts: Partner with Ayurvedic practitioners and experts to gain insights into traditional practices and the modern challenges they face.

Identify Gaps and Needs: Identify the gaps in the current diagnostic and treatment methods. This can include non-invasive diagnostic tools or software that can aid in personalized treatment plans.

Product Design and Development: Work on the design and development of diagnostic equipment or software. Ensure that they align with Ayurvedic principles and practices.

Regulatory Compliance: Ensure that your products comply with relevant medical device regulations and standards. This is crucial for safety and credibility.

Testing and Validation: Thoroughly test and validate your equipment and software to ensure their accuracy and efficacy.

Clinical Trials: Conduct clinical trials to demonstrate the effectiveness of your products. Collaborate with Ayurvedic clinics and practitioners for this purpose.

Marketing and Distribution: Develop a marketing strategy to promote your products. Partner with Ayurvedic clinics, hospitals, and practitioners for distribution.

User Training: Offer training and support to users of your equipment and software. Ayurvedic practitioners and technicians should be proficient in their use.

Continuous Improvement: Stay updated with the latest advancements in Ayurveda and technology. Continuously improve your products based on feedback and new discoveries.

Education and Awareness: Educate both practitioners and patients about the benefits and applications of your equipment and software.

Feedback and Adaptation: Collect feedback from users and be ready to adapt your products to meet evolving needs.

Remember, the development of equipment and software in the field of Ayurveda should be done with utmost respect for its traditional principles and a commitment to improving healthcare outcomes while preserving the authenticity of Ayurvedic practices.

*****

Chapter 10

Education Training and Events

बलमारोग्यमायुश्च प्राणाश्चाग्नौ प्रतिष्ठिताः|
अन्नपानेन्धनैश्चाग्निर्ज्वलति व्येति चान्यथा ||३४२||

Balamarogyamayushcha pranashchangnau

pratishthita,annapanendhanaishchagnirjwalati vyeti chanyatha

Strength, health, longevity and vital breath are dependent upon the power of digestion including metabolism. When supplied with fuel in the form of food and drinks, this power of digestion is sustained; it dwindles when deprived of it.

Charaka Sutra Sthana,Chapter 28, verse 342

HIGHLIGHTS

Establishing an Ayurvedic college, training institute and online Ayurveda certificate courses, involves regulatory compliance, qualified faculty, a comprehensive curriculum, infrastructure, financial planning, and long-term sustainability, with the need to balance profitability considerations alongside a commitment to Ayurvedic principles.

Unlock the business potential of Ayurveda by organizing events, conferences, and workshops that cater to the rising global interest in holistic health and wellness."

ESTABLISHING AYURVEDIC COLLEGES

Establishing Ayurvedic colleges as a business venture can be a complex undertaking with several considerations:

Regulations and Accreditation: Ensure that your college complies with all local and national regulations. Ayurvedic colleges often need accreditation from relevant authorities.

Qualified Faculty: Hire experienced and qualified Ayurvedic practitioners as faculty members to maintain educational standards.

Curriculum Development: Develop a comprehensive and up-to-date curriculum that covers traditional Ayurvedic practices, modern medicine, and business management for students.

Facilities and Infrastructure: Invest in proper infrastructure, classrooms, labs, and herbal gardens to facilitate hands-on learning.

Student Services: Provide academic and career support services to students, including placement assistance.

Marketing and Branding: Create a strong brand presence and marketing strategy to attract students.

Financial Planning: Carefully plan the finances, as it can be costly to set up and maintain an Ayurvedic college.

Sustainability: Consider how your college will remain financially viable over the long term.

Community Engagement: Build relationships with the local Ayurvedic community and healthcare organizations.

Compliance with Ayurvedic Principles: Ensure that the college adheres to the core principles of Ayurveda in teaching and practice.

It's crucial to have a deep understanding of Ayurveda and the education sector, as well as a passion for promoting Ayurvedic practices and healthcare. Consulting with experts and legal advisors can help ensure a successful and ethical venture.

The profitability of establishing an Ayurvedic college can vary significantly based on several factors, including location, competition, the quality of education, and the demand for Ayurvedic programs. Here are some considerations:

Location: The demand for Ayurvedic education can be higher in regions where Ayurveda is well-recognized and accepted. Urban areas may attract more students.

Competition: Assess the level of competition from existing Ayurvedic colleges and traditional medical institutions. Identifying a unique niche or specialization can help attract students.

Quality of Education: Providing high-quality education and experienced faculty can make your college more attractive to students.

Demand: Consider the local and global demand for Ayurvedic practitioners. Some regions may have a higher demand for holistic healthcare options.

Marketing and Outreach: Effective marketing and outreach efforts can influence the number of students enrolling in your college.

Long-Term Sustainability: It may take time to establish the college's reputation and gain recognition, so patience and a long-term perspective are important.

While Ayurveda is gaining popularity as an alternative form of medicine, financial success in establishing an Ayurvedic college may take time and may not be as immediately lucrative as other businesses. It's important to balance the financial aspect with a genuine commitment to promoting Ayurvedic principles and holistic healthcare. Conduct a detailed feasibility study and financial analysis to assess the potential return on investment for your specific location and circumstances.

Degree and Diplomas in ayurveda

Ayurveda is an ancient system of medicine that originated in India over 5,000 years ago. It is based on a holistic approach to healthcare, focusing on the balance between the body, mind, and spirit. In the field of Ayurveda, both degrees and diplomas play a crucial role in training and certifying practitioners.

Degrees In Ayurveda:

Bachelor of Ayurvedic Medicine and Surgery (BAMS): BAMS is a comprehensive undergraduate degree program in Ayurvedic medicine. It typically spans five and a half years and includes both theoretical and practical training. Graduates of BAMS are considered qualified Ayurvedic doctors and can diagnose, treat, and prescribe Ayurvedic remedies.

Doctor of Medicine (MD) in Ayurveda:

Post-graduation in Ayurveda, often referred to as MD (Doctor of Medicine) or MS (Master of Surgery), is offered in various specializations. Some common subjects for post-graduation in Ayurveda include:

Kayachikitsa (Internal Medicine)

Shalya Tantra (Surgery)

Shalakya Tantra (Ophthalmology and ENT)

Prasuti Tantra & Stri Roga (Obstetrics and Gynecology)

Kaumarabhritya (Pediatrics)

Panchakarma (Ayurvedic Detoxification and Rejuvenation)

Dravyaguna (Pharmacology and Materia Medica)

Rasa Shastra & Bhaishajya Kalpana (Ayurvedic Pharmaceutics)

Agada Tantra (Toxicology and Forensic Medicine)

Swasthavritta (Preventive and Social Medicine)

The availability of these specializations may vary between different Ayurvedic colleges and universities. It's essential to check with the specific institution or university for the specific post-graduate programs they offer.

Master of Science (MSc) in Ayurveda: MSc programs in Ayurveda focus on research and often include specialized areas of study. Graduates may work as researchers, educators, or consultants.

Diplomas in Ayurveda:

Diploma in Ayurvedic Nursing: This program is designed for those interested in nursing within an Ayurvedic healthcare setting. It covers patient care, traditional therapies, and herbal remedies.

Diploma in Panchakarma Therapy: Panchakarma is a purification and detoxification therapy in Ayurveda. This diploma program trains individuals in various Panchakarma techniques.

Diploma in Ayurvedic Pharmacy: This program focuses on the preparation and dispensing of Ayurvedic medicines. Graduates can work in Ayurvedic pharmacies or manufacturing units.

Diploma in Ayurvedic Wellness and Lifestyle Management: This diploma program educates students on the principles of Ayurveda for promoting wellness and a balanced lifestyle.

Both degrees and diplomas in Ayurveda are essential in promoting the practice and understanding of this traditional healing system. Degrees like BAMS provide a strong foundation for medical practice, while diplomas offer specialized knowledge in areas like therapy, pharmacy, and lifestyle management. As Ayurveda gains recognition worldwide, these educational paths ensure qualified professionals and practitioners who can contribute to the well-being of individuals through holistic healthcare.

CREATING AYURVEDA TRAINING INSTITUTES

Creating Ayurveda training institutes can be a promising business venture, but it requires careful planning and consideration of several factors:

Regulations and Licensing: Ensure that you comply with the legal and regulatory requirements for offering Ayurveda training. Different countries or regions may have specific guidelines for such institutes.

Curriculum and Instructors: Develop a comprehensive curriculum with experienced instructors who are well-versed in Ayurvedic principles and practices. High-quality education is crucial for the success of your institute.

Facilities: Create a conducive learning environment with well-equipped classrooms, herbal gardens, and practical training facilities.

Accreditation: Consider seeking accreditation or certification from relevant bodies to enhance the credibility of your institute.

Marketing and Promotion: Develop a marketing strategy to reach potential students. Highlight the benefits of Ayurveda training and what makes your institute stand out.

Financial Planning: Calculate the initial investment required, including staff salaries, infrastructure, and ongoing operational costs. Determine the pricing structure for your courses.

Partnerships: Collaborate with Ayurvedic practitioners, hospitals, or wellness centers to offer internships, practical experience, and job placement opportunities for your students.

Technology: Implement modern teaching technologies and e-learning platforms to enhance the learning experience.

Community Engagement: Engage with the local Ayurvedic community to build a network of support and resources.

Continuous Improvement: Stay updated with the latest developments in Ayurveda and education techniques, and be open to feedback from students for continuous improvement.

Remember that success may take time, and it's essential to be patient and persistent in building a reputable Ayurveda training institute.

DESIGNING ONLINE CERTIFICATE COURSES FOR AYURVEDA PRACTITIONERS AND GENERAL PUBLIC

Designing online certificate courses in Ayurveda can be a promising business venture. Here are the key steps to get started:

Market Research: Understand the demand for Ayurveda courses among practitioners and the general public. Identify your target audience and their specific needs.

Course Content: Develop comprehensive course content that covers Ayurvedic principles, practices, and therapies. Consider different levels of courses, from beginner to advanced.

Certification: Ensure that your courses provide valid certification upon completion. Collaborate with recognized Ayurveda institutions if possible.

Instructors: Hire experienced Ayurveda practitioners and educators to teach the courses. Their expertise will lend credibility to your program.

Platform Selection: Choose a reliable e-learning platform to host your courses. Ensure it supports video lectures, quizzes, assignments, and discussion forums.

Website and Branding: Create a professional website and branding that conveys trustworthiness and expertise in Ayurveda.

Marketing and Promotion: Develop a marketing strategy to reach your target audience. Utilize social media, email marketing, and partnerships with Ayurveda clinics or wellness centers.

Pricing: Set competitive pricing for your courses. Consider offering discounts for early adopters or bundled course packages.

Feedback and Improvement: Collect feedback from students and continuously improve your courses based on their input.

Legal and Regulatory Compliance: Ensure your courses comply with any legal or regulatory requirements for online education and Ayurveda practice.

Customer Support: Provide excellent customer support to assist students with any queries or technical issues.

Scaling: As your business grows, consider expanding your course offerings and reaching a global audience.

Remember that the quality of your courses and the credibility of your instructors are critical for success in the online education market. Ayurveda's growing popularity as an alternative healthcare system can make this venture profitable if executed well.

ORGANISING AYURVEDA CONFERENCES AND WORKSHOPS

In recent years, there has been a surge of

Interest in Ayurveda, creating significant business opportunities in the form of events, conferences, and workshops dedicated to this traditional science. Here we explore the potential for establishing and running such ventures in the field of Ayurveda.

THE RISING POPULARITY OF AYURVEDA

Ayurveda's popularity has been steadily increasing worldwide, thanks to its holistic approach to health and well-being. As individuals seek alternative and complementary methods to conventional medicine, Ayurveda has become a preferred choice for many. The increasing demand for Ayurvedic treatments, therapies, and products presents a lucrative business prospect for those involved in the field.

EVENTS, CONFERENCES, AND WORKSHOPS IN AYURVEDA

Events: Hosting Ayurveda-themed events, such as wellness retreats, yoga and Ayurveda workshops, or Ayurvedic food festivals, can attract participants interested in learning and experiencing the principles of Ayurveda. These events can generate revenue through ticket sales, sponsorships, and merchandise sales.

Conferences: Ayurvedic conferences bring together experts, practitioners, and enthusiasts to discuss the latest developments in Ayurveda. Organizing such events not only benefits the community but can also be financially rewarding through registration fees, exhibitor fees, and partnerships with Ayurvedic brands.

Workshops: Ayurveda workshops are an excellent way to educate and empower individuals to incorporate Ayurvedic practices into their daily lives. These workshops can cover topics like Ayurvedic cooking, yoga, or herbal remedies. Tuition fees for such workshops can be a source of income.

CHALLENGES AND CONSIDERATIONS

While the Ayurveda events and workshops business can be financially rewarding, several considerations and challenges need to be addressed:

Regulatory Compliance: Ensure compliance with local and international regulations concerning the practice and promotion of Ayurveda.

Quality and Authenticity: Maintaining the authenticity and quality of Ayurvedic content and treatments is essential to gain trust and credibility.

Marketing and Promotion: Effectively marketing your events, conferences, and workshops is crucial to attract participants and sponsors.

Competitive Landscape: The market for Ayurveda events is competitive. Identifying a niche or unique selling point is essential for success.

Conclusion: The rising global interest in Ayurveda offers a promising business opportunity for those passionate about holistic health and wellness. Events, conferences, and workshops in Ayurveda can serve as a viable business avenue, offering educational, experiential, and networking opportunities for enthusiasts while generating revenue. However, success in this venture requires careful planning, a commitment to quality and authenticity, and effective marketing strategies to stand out in a competitive market. By tapping into the growing demand for Ayurvedic knowledge and practices, entrepreneurs can contribute to the promotion and expansion of this ancient system of medicine while building a profitable business.

*****

Chapter 11

Publishing and Digital Media In Ayurveda

वर्तयन्ति प्रीणिताः सर्वदेहिनः ।
यद्दते सर्वभूतानां जीवितं नावतिष्ठते॥९॥

Vartyanti pidhitaah sarvadehinah,yadhyte
sarvbhutaanaam jivitam na-avtishthete

Ojas keeps all living beings nourished and refreshed.

There can be no life without Ojas.

Ojas is a quantifiable liquid in the body, responsible for overall health, energy and liveliness. It is both a mental and physical factor, the essence of all the body tissues.

Charaka Sutra Sthana, Chapter 30, verse 9

HIGHLIGHTS

Create Ayurveda content through books, eBooks, and magazines by deepening your knowledge, identifying your niche, writing well-researched content, and promoting it while staying updated and authentic.

Developing as an Ayurveda YouTuber and blogger involves education, niche selection, high-quality content creation, branding, SEO optimization, audience interaction, and patience in building a dedicated community.

CREATE AYURVEDA CONTENT THROUGH BOOKS, E BOOKS, MAGAZINES

Creating Ayurveda content through books, eBooks, and magazines can be a rewarding way to share knowledge about this ancient system of medicine. Here's a brief outline of how you can go about it:

Research and Study: Start by deepening your understanding of Ayurveda. Read classical Ayurvedic texts, modern interpretations, and research articles to gain comprehensive knowledge.

Identify Your Niche: Ayurveda is a vast field. Decide on a specific niche or aspect of Ayurveda that you are passionate about, whether it's herbal remedies, diet, yoga, or Ayurvedic lifestyle practices.

WRITING YOUR CONTENT

Books: Write a comprehensive book on your chosen Ayurvedic niche. Ensure its well-researched, organized, and accessible to a broad audience.

eBooks: Consider creating shorter, more focused eBooks that can be easily distributed online. These can delve into specific topics or remedies.

Magazine Articles: Write articles that are suitable for magazine publication, typically shorter and more general. Magazines often prefer pieces that are engaging and practical.

PUBLISHING AND FORMATTING:

For books, consider traditional publishing or self-publishing on platforms like Amazon Kindle.

For eBooks, format them in a user-friendly manner and distribute through platforms like Amazon Kindle, Apple Books, or your website.

For magazine articles, research publications that are interested in Ayurveda content and submit your work following their guidelines.

PROMOTION:

Use social media, blogs, and websites to promote your content. Establish yourself as an Ayurveda expert and engage with your audience.

Collaborate with Ayurveda practitioners or experts for endorsements or joint projects.

Attend relevant events and conferences to network and promote your work.

Stay Updated: Ayurveda is an evolving field. Keep yourself updated with the latest research and developments to ensure your content remains relevant.

Compliance and Authenticity: Ensure that the information you provide is accurate and adheres to ethical standards. Ayurveda is a complex field, and misinformation can be harmful.

Feedback and Iteration: Be open to feedback and improve your content over time. Listen to your audience's needs and adapt accordingly.

Remember that creating Ayurveda content should be a labor of love, driven by a genuine passion for this ancient system of medicine and a commitment to sharing its wisdom with others.

DEVELOP YOURSELF AS AYURVEDA YOUTUBER AND BLOGGER

To develop yourself as an Ayurveda YouTuber and blogger, you can follow these steps:

EDUCATION AND CERTIFICATION

Obtain formal education or certification in Ayurveda to establish your credibility.

NICHE SELECTION

Choose a specific niche within Ayurveda that you are passionate about, such as Ayurveda medicinal treatment, herbal remedies, diet and nutrition, yoga, or lifestyle practices.

CONTENT PLANNING

Develop a content strategy that outlines the topics you want to cover and the value you can provide to your audience.

CREATE HIGH-QUALITY CONTENT

Produce well-researched, informative, and engaging videos and blog posts. Invest in good recording equipment and editing software.

CONSISTENCY

Maintain a regular posting schedule to keep your audience engaged and informed.

BRANDING

Develop a unique and recognizable brand for your channel and blog, including a logo, color scheme, and consistent branding across all platforms.

SEO OPTIMIZATION

Optimize your content for search engines to reach a wider audience. Use relevant keywords and meta descriptions.

INTERACT WITH YOUR AUDIENCE

Respond to comments and engage with your viewers on social media platforms to build a community.

COLLABORATIONS

Collaborate with other Ayurveda practitioners or You Tubers to expand your reach.

MONETIZATION

Explore different monetization options like ads, affiliate marketing, sponsored content, and merchandise sales.

STAY UPDATED

Keep yourself updated on the latest developments in Ayurveda and related fields to provide accurate and up-to-date information.

NETWORKING

Attend Ayurveda conferences, webinars, and workshops to network with experts and stay connected with the Ayurveda community.

LEGAL CONSIDERATIONS

Be aware of any legal and ethical considerations in your content, especially when discussing medical topics.

PATIENCE AND PERSISTENCE

Building a successful YouTube channel and blog takes time. Be patient and persistent in your efforts.

ANALYTICS

Use analytics tools to track the performance of your content and adjust your strategy accordingly.

HEALTH AND WELL-BEING

Since you're focusing on Ayurveda, prioritize your own health and well-being to be a good example to your audience.

Remember that it might take time to build an audience, but by consistently providing valuable content and connecting with your viewers, you can grow as an Ayurveda You Tuber and blogger.

DIGITAL AYURVEDA HEALTH PLATFORM

In an era of rapid technological advancement, the healthcare industry has witnessed significant transformation. One noteworthy development is the emergence of digital platforms that bridge traditional medical practices with modern technology. The Digital Ayurveda Health Platform is a pioneering example, fusing the ancient wisdom of Ayurveda with digital innovation to provide holistic health solutions. This essay explores the evolution, features, benefits, and challenges of this revolutionary platform.

EVOLUTION OF DIGITAL AYURVEDA HEALTH PLATFORMS

Ayurveda, an ancient system of medicine with roots in India, has long been valued for its holistic approach to healthcare. Traditional Ayurvedic treatments consider an individual's physical, mental, and spiritual well-being. However, the integration of Ayurveda into the digital realm is relatively recent. The evolution of Digital Ayurveda Health Platforms can be traced to the growing awareness of alternative medicine, wellness trends, and the desire for personalized healthcare solutions.

KEY FEATURES OF DIGITAL AYURVEDA HEALTH PLATFORMS

Personalized Wellness Plans: These platforms leverage artificial intelligence and data analysis to create customized wellness plans based on an individual's constitution (Prakriti) and current health status.

Telemedicine and Consultations: Users can consult experienced Ayurvedic practitioners through video calls, chat, or voice calls, offering accessibility to Ayurvedic healthcare from the comfort of their homes.

Lifestyle and Diet Recommendations: Digital Ayurveda platforms provide guidance on suitable diets, exercise routines, and daily practices according to Ayurvedic principles.

Herbal Medicine Suggestions: Based on an individual's health needs, Ayurvedic platforms recommend herbal remedies and supplements.

Health Monitoring: Users can track their health progress and receive regular updates on their wellness journey through the platform.

BENEFITS OF DIGITAL AYURVEDA HEALTH PLATFORMS

Holistic Care: These platforms offer a comprehensive approach to health, addressing physical, mental, and spiritual well-being.

Accessibility: Users can access Ayurvedic consultations and recommendations from anywhere, reducing geographical barriers.

Personalization: Tailored wellness plans ensure that each individual's unique needs are met.

Integration with Modern Medicine: These platforms can complement conventional medical treatments, providing a holistic approach to healing.

Empowerment: Users are actively involved in their health management, making informed choices about their well-being.

CHALLENGES AND CONCERNS

Quality Control: Ensuring the authenticity and quality of Ayurvedic advice and products provided online is a significant challenge.

Data Privacy: Protecting user health data and maintaining patient-doctor confidentiality is crucial.

Lack of Regulation: The absence of standardized guidelines and regulations for Ayurvedic digital platforms can lead to variations in quality and safety.

Cultural Sensitivity: Ensuring that Ayurveda is understood and practiced in a culturally sensitive and respectful manner is vital, especially in cross-cultural settings.

Conclusion: Digital Ayurveda Health Platforms represent a promising convergence of ancient wisdom and modern technology, offering holistic healthcare solutions to a global audience. These platforms provide accessibility, personalization, and empowerment, enhancing the overall wellness experience. However, addressing challenges related to quality control, data privacy, regulation, and cultural sensitivity is imperative to ensure that these platforms continue to be a valuable addition to the healthcare landscape. As technology continues to evolve, the Digital Ayurveda Health Platform is poised to play a vital role in shaping the future of healthcare.

*****

Section-3

Building and Scaling Your Ayurveda Venture

Chapter 12

Starting Your Ayurveda Venture

परुषस्यातिमात्रस्यसूचकस्यानृतस्यच|

वाक्यस्याकालयुक्तस्य धारयेद्वेगमुत्थितम्||२८|

Parushyatimaatrasya suchakasyaanratasya cha,
vakyasyaakaalyuktasya dharyedwagamuthitam

In speaking, one should suppress the urges of…

Parusha – speaking extremely harsh words,

Atimatra – speaking excessively,

Soochaka – backbiting,

Anruta – lies,

Akala Vakya – use of untimely words.

-Charaka Sutra Sthana,Chapter 7, verse 28

HIGHLIGHTS

Launch your Ayurveda venture successfully by focusing on market research, compliance, customer experience, and sustainable growth, all while emphasizing the holistic nature of Ayurvedic healthcare.

Promote Ayurvedic products and services effectively by combining traditional and digital marketing strategies, while prioritizing ethics and customer well-being.

STEPS TO LAUNCH YOUR AYURVEDA VENTURE

Launching an Ayurveda venture involves several steps:

Market Research:

Identify your target audience and their healthcare needs.

Analyze the competitive landscape in your area.

Business Plan:

Create a detailed business plan outlining your venture's goals, services, and budget.

Legal Requirements:

Register your business and obtain the necessary licenses and permits.

Comply with regulations related to Ayurvedic products and services.

Location:

Choose a suitable location for your Ayurveda clinic or store.

Product/Service Offering:

Decide on the Ayurvedic products or services you'll provide.

Source quality Ayurvedic products or hire trained practitioners.

Branding and Marketing:

Develop a brand identity and marketing strategy.

Create a website and establish a strong online presence.

Use social media and content marketing to reach your target audience.

Staffing:

Hire qualified Ayurvedic practitioners and support staff.

Ensure they are certified and knowledgeable in Ayurveda.

Customer Experience:

Focus on providing an excellent customer experience.

Educate customers about the benefits of Ayurveda.

Pricing and Financial Management:

Determine your pricing strategy.

Set up an accounting system and manage finances effectively.

Partnerships and Networking:

Build relationships with local healthcare providers and complementary businesses.

Join Ayurveda associations and attend relevant events.

Compliance and Quality:

Follow all Ayurvedic principles and maintain product quality.

Stay informed about updates in Ayurvedic practices.

Launch and Promotion:

Host an opening event or launch campaign to attract customers.

Offer promotions or discounts in the initial phase.

Customer Feedback and Improvement:

Gather feedback from customers to improve your services.

Adapt to changing customer needs and market trends.

Sustainability and Growth:

Plan for long-term sustainability and growth.

Consider expanding to multiple locations or offering online consultations.

Continuous Learning:

Stay updated on Ayurvedic research and practices.

Invest in ongoing education for your team.

Remember that Ayurveda is a holistic approach to healthcare, so emphasize the importance of personalized treatment and wellness. Be patient and persistent, as building a successful Ayurveda venture can take time.

FUNDING AND INVESTMENT STRATEGIES FOR STARTING AYURVEDA VENTURE

Starting an Ayurveda venture can be a rewarding endeavor, but it requires careful planning, funding, and investment strategies. Here are some steps to consider:

Business Plan: Start by creating a detailed business plan that outlines your vision, mission, target market, products or services, and financial projections. This plan will be essential for attracting investors and securing funding.

Self-Financing: Consider using your own savings or personal investments to kickstart the venture. This shows your commitment and dedication to potential investors.

Seek Investors: Look for investors who are interested in the healthcare or wellness sector. You can approach angel investors, venture capitalists, or even crowdfunding platforms that specialize in healthcare and wellness projects.

Grants and Government Programs: Research if there are any grants or government programs that support traditional medicine and wellness initiatives. Many governments promote the growth of such industries.

Bank Loans: You can explore the option of taking out a bank loan or seeking financing from financial institutions. Make sure to have a strong business plan and collateral if needed.

Partnerships: Consider forming strategic partnerships with existing healthcare providers or wellness centers. This can help reduce initial investment and leverage their existing customer base.

Bootstrapping: Start small and gradually reinvest profits into the business. This method allows for organic growth without relying on external investors.

Market Research: Conduct through market research to understand the demand for Ayurveda products and services in your target area. This will help you make informed investment decisions.

Quality Assurance: Allocate funds for quality control and assurance to ensure that your products or services meet regulatory standards and customer expectations.

Marketing and Branding: Invest in effective marketing and branding strategies to promote your Ayurveda venture. This will help attract customers and generate revenue.

Professional Advice: Consult with legal and financial experts who have experience in healthcare and wellness businesses. They can provide valuable guidance on funding and investment strategies specific to your venture.

Regulatory Compliance: Be aware of the regulatory requirements for Ayurveda products and services. Allocate funds for compliance and any necessary certifications.

Remember that the success of your Ayurveda venture depends on a combination of funding, a solid business strategy, and the ability to provide high-quality products or services that meet the needs of your target market.

BUILD A TRUSTED BRAND IN AYURVEDA

Building a trusted brand in the field of Ayurveda, or any industry, involves several key steps:

Authenticity and Quality: Ensure that your Ayurvedic products or services are of the highest quality and are based on authentic Ayurvedic principles. This may involve sourcing high-quality ingredients, using traditional preparation methods, and adhering to Ayurvedic standards.

Transparency: Be transparent about your products, their ingredients, and the processes you use. Clear and accurate labeling is essential. This helps build trust with your customers.

Certifications and Compliance: Obtain relevant certifications and comply with regulatory requirements. This could include certifications from Ayurvedic governing bodies and adherence to safety and quality standards.

Expertise: Employ or consult with experts in Ayurveda. Having knowledgeable practitioners or advisors can help ensure your products or services are based on sound Ayurvedic principles.

Customer Education: Educate your customers about Ayurveda and your products. Provide information on how Ayurveda works, the benefits of your products, and how they should be used. Knowledgeable customers are more likely to trust your brand.

Ethical Marketing: Avoid making exaggerated claims or promises. Ethical marketing builds trust. Provide real testimonials and share the science behind your products.

Customer Feedback: Encourage and act upon customer feedback. Listen to their concerns, make improvements, and show that you value their input.

Consistency: Consistency in product quality and service is crucial. Customers should be able to trust that your products will perform as expected every time.

Community Engagement: Engage with the Ayurvedic community. Participate in events, seminars, and discussions related to Ayurveda. This helps establish your brand within the community.

Online Presence: Establish a strong online presence, including a professional website and social media profiles. Use these platforms to share valuable content and engage with your audience.

Distribution and Availability: Ensure your products are readily available and accessible. Widespread availability contributes to trust as customers can easily find your products.

Customer Support: Provide excellent customer support. Address customer inquiries and issues promptly and professionally.

Sustainability: If applicable, incorporate sustainable and eco-friendly practices into your brand. Modern consumers often trust brands that are environmentally conscious.

Long-Term Commitment: Building trust takes time. Be committed to long-term growth and improvement. Trust is often built over years of consistent and reliable performance.

Legal Protection: Protect your brand through trademarks and legal means. This can help prevent unauthorized use of your brand name and products.

Remember that building trust is an ongoing process. It requires dedication, authenticity, and a commitment to delivering value to your customers within the framework of Ayurveda.

PROMOTING PRODUCT AND SERVICES

Promoting Ayurvedic products and services can be done effectively through a combination of traditional and digital marketing strategies. Here are some steps to help you get started:

Understand Ayurveda: Gain a deep understanding of Ayurveda and its principles. This will help you communicate the benefits of your products and services more effectively.

Quality Assurance: Ensure that your products are of high quality and comply with relevant regulations. This builds trust with your customers.

Website and Online Presence: Create a professional website to showcase your products and services. Use social media platforms to engage with your audience.

Content Marketing: Share valuable content related to Ayurveda through blogs, articles, videos, and info graphics. This positions you as an authority in the field.

Search Engine Optimization (SEO): Optimize your website and content for search engines to improve your online visibility.

Social Media Marketing: Use platforms like Instagram, Facebook, and Twitter to share educational content, customer testimonials, and engage with your audience.

Email Marketing: Build an email list and send newsletters with information about Ayurvedic practices, product updates, and special offers.

Collaborate with Influencers: Partner with Ayurveda experts or influencers who can endorse your products and services.

Local Marketing: If you have a physical location, promote your services through local advertising, such as flyers and local SEO.

Customer Reviews and Testimonials: Encourage satisfied customers to leave reviews on your website or on relevant platforms. Positive reviews can boost your credibility.

Educational Workshops: Organize workshops, webinars, or seminars to educate people about Ayurveda and your offerings.

Networking: Attend Ayurvedic conferences and network with professionals in the field to expand your reach.

Loyalty Programs: Create loyalty programs or offer discounts to repeat customers.

Traditional Marketing: Use print media, such as brochures, posters, and newspapers, if your target audience responds well to these methods.

Compliance and Ethics: Ensure that your marketing materials and practices adhere to ethical standards and are in compliance with Ayurvedic principles and local regulations.

Feedback and Improvement: Continuously seek feedback from your customers to improve your products and services.

Remember that promoting Ayurvedic products and services should be done ethically and with a focus on improving the health and well-being of your customers. Always prioritize their safety and provide accurate information.

HOW TO SCALE YOUR AYURVEDA VENTURE

Scaling an Ayurveda venture involves careful planning and execution. Here are some ways to scale your Ayurveda business:

Diversify Product Line: Expand your range of Ayurvedic products, including herbal supplements, skincare, haircare, and wellness products.

Online Presence: Develop a strong online presence through a website and social media to reach a wider audience.

E-commerce: Sell your products through e-commerce platforms to access a global customer base.

Franchising: Consider franchising your Ayurveda clinic or store to reach different geographic locations.

Collaborations: Partner with established Ayurvedic practitioners, yoga centers, or wellness spas to offer integrated services.

Quality Assurance: Maintain high-quality standards and certifications to build trust among customers.

Educational Programs: Offer Ayurveda courses and workshops to train new practitioners and expand your reach.

Exporting: Explore international markets by exporting your Ayurvedic products.

Research and Development: Invest in research to develop new Ayurvedic formulations and improve existing ones.

Marketing and Branding: Invest in marketing to create a strong brand identity and reach a larger audience.

Digital Marketing: Use online advertising, content marketing, and search engine optimization to increase visibility.

Customer Feedback: Continuously gather and act on customer feedback to improve your products and services.

Leverage Technology: Implement technology solutions for inventory management, customer relations, and online consultations.

Regulatory Compliance: Ensure compliance with local and international regulations for Ayurvedic products.

Health and Wellness Centers: Open holistic wellness centers that provide Ayurvedic treatments, yoga, and meditation.

Strategic Alliances: Partner with other wellness or health-related businesses to cross-promote services.

Investor Funding: Seek funding from investors to accelerate growth and expansion.

Community Engagement: Engage with the Ayurveda community and collaborate on research and knowledge sharing.

Customer Loyalty Programs: Create loyalty programs and incentives to retain existing customers.

Sustainable Practices: Emphasize eco-friendly and sustainable practices to appeal to environmentally conscious consumers.

Remember that scaling should be a gradual process, and it's essential to maintain the quality and authenticity of Ayurvedic practices while expanding your venture.

*****

Chapter 13

Regulatory Framework

लोभशोकभयक्रोधमानवेगान् विधारयेत्।
नैर्लज्ज्येर्ष्यातिरागाणामभिध्यायाश्च बुद्धिमान्॥२७॥

Lobhshokbhyakrodhamaanvegaan vidharyet,
nirlajjyeshyartiraganambhidhyaayaashcha buddhiman

A wise person should suppress mental urges pertaining to the following.

Lobha – greed

Shoka – grief

Bhaya – fear

Krodha – anger

Mana – vanity

Nairlajja – shamelessness

Irshya – jealousy

Atiraga – excessive desire

Abhidhyaya – ill will, malice

Charaka Sutra Sthana,Chapter 7, verse 27

HIGHLIGHTS

Regulation of Ayurveda practice and trade in India is governed by the Ministry of AYUSH while international recognition and standards differ by country, to country making it essential to research local regulations.

Compliance and quality control in Ayurveda are pivotal for ensuring the safety and efficacy of products and treatments, encompassing regulatory adherence, ingredient quality, testing, and ethical standards.

AYURVEDA REGULATIONS IN INDIA AND WORLDWIDE

Regulation of Ayurveda practice and trade in India and worldwide varies significantly. Here, I'll provide an overview of the regulatory framework for Ayurveda in both contexts.

REGULATION IN INDIA

National Commission for Indian System of Medicine (NCISM) In India, a statutory body under the Ministry of AYUSH (Ayurveda, Yoga and Naturopathy, Unani, Siddha, and Homoeopathy). The NCISM sets standards for education and practice of Ayurveda.

Education and Licensing: Ayurvedic practitioners must complete a Bachelor of Ayurvedic Medicine and Surgery (BAMS) degree from a recognized institution. After graduation, they may register with state medical councils to practice legally. India has a robust system of Ayurvedic colleges and universities.

Ayurvedic Drugs and Pharmaceuticals: The manufacture, sale, and distribution of Ayurvedic medicines are regulated by the Drugs and Cosmetics Act, 1940. The Ayurvedic Pharmacopoeia of India contains standards for these medicines.

Ayurvedic Clinical Practice: Registered Ayurvedic doctors can diagnose and treat patients using Ayurvedic principles and medicines. However, they are not authorized to perform modern surgical procedures or prescribe allopathic drugs.

REGULATION WORLDWIDE

Recognition Varies: The recognition and regulation of Ayurveda differ widely outside of India. In some countries, Ayurveda is recognized and integrated into the healthcare system, while in others, it's considered an alternative or complementary therapy.

Licensing and Education: In countries where Ayurveda is regulated, practitioners may be required to meet specific educational and licensing standards. These standards vary significantly from one nation to another.

Safety and Quality Control: In countries where Ayurvedic products are available, there may be regulations to ensure the safety and quality of Ayurvedic medicines and treatments. Some nations have their own pharmacopoeias for Ayurvedic products.

Integration into Healthcare Systems: In some countries, Ayurveda is integrated into the healthcare system, and Ayurvedic treatments are offered alongside conventional medicine. In others, Ayurveda is considered a complementary or alternative therapy.

Certification Bodies: Several international organizations and councils certify Ayurvedic practitioners and promote standardization and quality control.

It's essential to research the specific regulations and standards in the country where you plan to practice or receive Ayurvedic treatments. Ayurveda's status and acceptance as a legitimate medical system can vary greatly, and understanding the local regulatory framework is crucial for safe and effective practice and trade.

COMPLIANCE AND QUALITY CONTROL IN AYURVEDA

Compliance and quality control in Ayurveda are essential to ensure the safety and efficacy of Ayurvedic products and treatments. Here are some key points to consider:

Regulatory Framework: Ayurveda is regulated in many countries, including India, through specific regulatory bodies and guidelines. Compliance with these regulations is crucial to ensure that Ayurvedic products meet safety and quality standards.

Quality Control of Ingredients: Ayurvedic treatments often use herbs and natural ingredients. It's important to ensure the quality and authenticity of these ingredients through proper sourcing, testing, and certification.

Good Manufacturing Practices (GMP): Ayurvedic product manufacturers should follow GMP standards to maintain consistency and quality during the manufacturing process.

Testing and Analysis: Regular testing of Ayurvedic medicines and products for contaminants, heavy metals, and other impurities is necessary. This includes analytical methods like High-Performance Liquid Chromatography (HPLC) to check the composition.

Documentation and Labeling: Proper documentation of formulations, manufacturing processes, and labeling is vital to demonstrate compliance with regulatory requirements.

Safety and Efficacy Studies: Research and clinical studies are essential to establish the safety and efficacy of Ayurvedic treatments. Compliance with ethical standards in research is crucial.

Ethical Practices: Ayurvedic practitioners should adhere to ethical standards and codes of conduct in their treatment methods.

Education and Training: Practitioners and manufacturers should receive proper education and training to ensure they have the necessary knowledge and skills to maintain compliance and quality.

Consumer Awareness: Educating consumers about Ayurvedic treatments, their proper use, and potential risks is essential to promote responsible use.

International Standards: For Ayurvedic products intended for export, compliance with international quality standards may be necessary.

Overall, ensuring compliance and quality control in Ayurveda is a multidimensional process that involves regulation, testing, documentation, and education to maintain the safety and effectiveness of Ayurvedic treatments and products

*****

Chapter 14

Ecofriendly Ayurveda

लाघवं कर्मसामर्थ्यं स्थैर्यं दुःखसहिष्णुता ।

दोषक्षयोऽग्निवृद्धिश्च व्यायामादुपजायते॥३२॥

Laghavam karmasaamarthyam sthyaram dukhasahishnutaa, doshakshyoagnivriddhishcha vyayamadupjaayate

The right amount of exercise brings about…

Laghavam – lightness in the body (and mind),

Karmasaamrthyam – an increase in work capacity,

Sthairyam – an increase in body stability,

Dukha sahishunta – improvement in resistance to discomfort,

Doshakshaya – a balance of the Tridosha,

Agnivruddhi – improvement in strength of digestion.

Charaka Sutra Sthana, Chapter 16, verse 32

HIGHLIGHTS

Integrating sustainable practices into your Ayurveda venture ensures eco-conscious and responsible operations while respecting Ayurvedic principles.

Sustainable Ayurveda integrates eco-friendly practices, ethical sourcing, and traditional knowledge preservation to harmonize well-being for individuals and the planet.

ENVIRONMENTAL CONSIDERATION FOR AYURVEDA VENTURE

Starting an Ayurveda venture comes with several environmental considerations to ensure sustainability and responsible practices:

Sustainable Sourcing: Ensure that herbs, plants, and ingredients used in Ayurvedic products are sourced sustainably to avoid overharvesting and habitat destruction.

Biodiversity Protection: Promote the conservation of biodiversity by using cultivated herbs or supporting responsible wild harvesting practices.

Organic Farming: Encourage organic farming practices to minimize the use of synthetic pesticides and fertilizers, which can harm the environment.

Waste Reduction: Minimize packaging waste by using eco-friendly and recyclable materials. Implement recycling and waste reduction programs within the venture.

Energy Efficiency: Adopt energy-efficient technologies and practices in production, distribution, and daily operations to reduce the carbon footprint.

Water Conservation: Implement water-saving measures in processing and consider the water footprint of products.

Eco-friendly Manufacturing: Use sustainable manufacturing processes and non-toxic materials to produce Ayurvedic products.

Transportation: Opt for eco-friendly transportation options for product distribution, reducing emissions.

Eco-certifications: Consider obtaining certifications like organic, Fair Trade, or other relevant eco-certifications to demonstrate commitment to environmental responsibility.

Education and Awareness: Educate employees and customers about environmental issues and promote sustainable living.

Waste Management: Properly manage waste, including disposal and recycling of herbal remnants and other byproducts.

Local Sourcing: Whenever possible, source ingredients locally to reduce the environmental impact of transportation.

Research and Innovation: Invest in research to develop environmentally friendly Ayurvedic formulations and products.

By integrating these environmental considerations into your Ayurveda venture, you can contribute to a more sustainable and eco-conscious business model while respecting the principles of Ayurveda.

SUSTAINABLE AYURVEDA

In recent years, there has been a growing emphasis on the importance of sustainability in various aspects of life, including healthcare. Sustainable Ayurveda refers to the practice of Ayurvedic medicine in a manner that is environmentally responsible, socially equitable, and economically viable. This essay explores the principles and practices of sustainable Ayurveda, highlighting its significance in promoting both individual well-being and the health of the planet.

PRINCIPLES OF SUSTAINABLE AYURVEDA

Eco-friendly Medicinal Plant Cultivation: Sustainable Ayurveda places great importance on the ethical and sustainable sourcing of medicinal herbs and plants. This involves promoting organic farming, avoiding overharvesting, and protecting endangered species. It encourages the cultivation of medicinal plants in a manner that respects biodiversity and natural ecosystems.

Preservation of Traditional Knowledge: Ayurveda relies on centuries-old wisdom and practices passed down through generations. Sustainable Ayurveda emphasizes the preservation of this traditional knowledge, ensuring that it is not lost or exploited. It also encourages the collaboration between traditional healers and modern researchers to validate the efficacy of Ayurvedic treatments.

Minimal Environmental Impact: Ayurvedic preparations often use natural substances, but it's crucial to ensure that the extraction and manufacturing processes have a minimal environmental footprint. Sustainable Ayurveda promotes the use of eco-friendly practices in the production of Ayurvedic medicines and cosmetics, including efficient waste management and energy conservation.

Ethical and Fair Trade: Sustainable Ayurveda supports fair trade practices, ensuring that local communities and farmers receive just compensation for their contributions to the industry. This approach not only promotes social equity but also encourages the sustainable growth of Ayurvedic resources.

Wellness beyond Physical Health: Ayurveda focuses on the holistic well-being of an individual, encompassing mental, emotional, and spiritual health. Sustainable Ayurveda integrates these dimensions, emphasizing the importance of mental and emotional equilibrium for sustainable living and personal well-being.

THE SIGNIFICANCE OF SUSTAINABLE AYURVEDA

Environmental Conservation: By promoting responsible harvesting and cultivation of medicinal plants, Sustainable Ayurveda contributes to the preservation of natural ecosystems and biodiversity. This ensures the continued availability of essential herbs for future generations.

Human Health and Wellness: Sustainable Ayurveda recognizes the interconnection between environmental health and human health. By encouraging eco-friendly practices, it fosters a healthier environment, which, in turn, promotes human well-being.

Cultural Heritage Preservation: Sustainable Ayurveda safeguards the rich cultural heritage of traditional healing practices. It respects the knowledge and wisdom of indigenous communities while integrating modern research and technology to enhance the effectiveness of Ayurvedic treatments.

Economic Viability: Sustainable Ayurveda encourages a balanced and sustainable business model for Ayurvedic practitioners and manufacturers. By avoiding overexploitation and ensuring fair trade, it supports the economic viability of the Ayurvedic industry.

Conclusion: Sustainable Ayurveda is a vital approach that harmonizes the principles of Ayurvedic medicine with environmental responsibility and social equity. By promoting eco-friendly practices, ethical sourcing, and the preservation of traditional knowledge, it ensures the well-being of both individuals and the planet. As the world continues to embrace sustainability, integrating these principles into the practice and propagation of Ayurveda is a promising way forward for the well-being of humanity and the Earth.

*****

Chapter 15

Future of Ayurveda

सत्त्वमात्मा शरीरं च त्रयमेतत्त्रिदण्डवत्|
लोकस्तिष्ठति संयोगात्तत्र सर्वं प्रतिष्ठितम्||४६||

Satvaatma shaariram cha tryametatridandvat,
lokastishthati sayogaattra sarvam pratishthitam

The tripods of life are *satva* (mind), *atma* (soul) and *shareera* (body). The world is sustained by their combination. They constitute the basis for everything.

Charaka Sutra Sthana, Chapter 1, verse 46

HIGHLIGHTS

Emerging trends in Ayurveda encompass integration with modern medicine, personalized wellness plans, Ayurvedic beauty products, yoga integration, digital accessibility, wellness tourism, herbal medicine adoption, mental health support, and a focus on research and standardization, ensuring its continued relevance in modern healthcare.

Technology has modernized Ayurveda, improving research, diagnosis, herbal medicine, telemedicine, and patient care through digitization and innovative tools.

EMERGING TRENDS IN AYURVEDA

Ayurveda, the ancient system of medicine that originated in India, has been gaining increased recognition and popularity in recent years. As people seek more holistic and natural approaches to healthcare, Ayurveda has witnessed several emerging trends that are shaping its future. These trends encompass various aspects of Ayurveda, including its practices, products, and integration into modern healthcare systems.

Integration with Modern Medicine: One of the most significant emerging trends is the integration of Ayurveda with modern medicine. Many healthcare institutions are recognizing the value of Ayurvedic principles and therapies in complementing conventional treatments. This trend aims to create a more comprehensive and patient-centric approach to healthcare by combining the strengths of both systems.

Personalized Ayurveda: Ayurveda has always emphasized the uniqueness of each individual's constitution, known as "Prakriti." Emerging trends in Ayurveda focus on personalized wellness plans tailored to a person's specific constitution and health needs. This approach incorporates personalized diets, herbal formulations, and lifestyle recommendations.

Ayurvedic Beauty and Skincare: The beauty and skincare industry has witnessed a surge in Ayurvedic products. Natural and herbal ingredients, as per Ayurvedic principles, are being incorporated into cosmetics and skincare products. This trend aligns with the broader movement towards clean and organic beauty products.

Yoga and Ayurveda Integration: Yoga and Ayurveda are closely related systems. An emerging trend involves the integration of yoga and Ayurveda to promote holistic well-being. Practitioners are encouraged to combine yoga postures, breathing exercises, and meditation with Ayurvedic dietary and lifestyle practices for better health.

Digital Ayurveda: The digital age has also impacted Ayurveda. Online platforms and mobile apps provide information, consultations, and even personalized treatment plans. These digital tools make Ayurveda more accessible and convenient for a global audience.

Ayurveda Tourism: Ayurvedic wellness retreats and tourism have gained popularity. Travelers seek rejuvenation through traditional Ayurvedic therapies, detoxification, and yoga in beautiful settings. This trend combines tourism with wellness and cultural experiences.

Herbal Medicine and Nutraceuticals: Ayurvedic herbs and formulations are finding their place in the nutraceutical and herbal medicine industries. Ayurvedic supplements are becoming popular choices for those looking for natural alternatives to conventional pharmaceuticals.

Ayurveda for Mental Health: Ayurveda's holistic approach extends to mental health. There's a growing interest in using Ayurvedic practices, such as meditation, stress management, and specific herbal remedies, to support mental and emotional well-being.

Research and Standardization: Ayurveda is evolving with a focus on research and standardization. Scientific studies are being conducted to validate the efficacy and safety of Ayurvedic treatments. This trend aims to bridge the gap between traditional knowledge and modern evidence-based medicine.

In conclusion, Ayurveda is experiencing a renaissance, with emerging trends that cater to the evolving needs and preferences of individuals seeking holistic health and well-being solutions. These trends ensure that Ayurveda continues to be a valuable and relevant healthcare system in the modern world, offering a unique blend of tradition and science.

ROLE OF TECHNOLOGY IN AYURVEDA

Technology has been playing an increasingly important role in Ayurveda, the traditional system of medicine from India. Here are some ways in which technology has influenced and enhanced Ayurveda:

Research and Documentation: Technology has enabled the digitization and preservation of ancient Ayurvedic texts, making them more accessible for study and research. This has led to a better understanding of Ayurvedic principles and practices.

Diagnosis and Assessment: Modern diagnostic tools, such as MRI, CT scans, and blood tests, are often used in conjunction with Ayurvedic diagnostic methods to provide a more comprehensive assessment of a patient's health.

Herbal Medicine: Technology has facilitated the identification, extraction, and standardization of herbal medicines used in Ayurveda. This ensures quality control and safety in the production of Ayurvedic remedies.

Telemedicine: Ayurvedic practitioners can now offer telemedicine services, allowing them to reach a broader patient base and provide consultations remotely. This has become especially relevant in the context of the COVID-19 pandemic.

Ayurveda Software: There are software tools designed for Ayurvedic practitioners to manage patient records, create treatment plans, and access reference materials, which streamline their practice.

Research and Data Analysis: Ayurvedic research is benefiting from data analytics and AI, which can help identify patterns and correlations in patient data to improve treatment outcomes.

Ayurveda and Wearable Devices: Integration with wearable devices and health apps allows individuals to track their health parameters, making it easier to align Ayurvedic practices with personal well-being goals.

Education and Outreach: Technology has made Ayurvedic knowledge more accessible to a global audience through online courses, webinars, and educational apps.

Quality Control: Technology is used to ensure the quality of Ayurvedic products, such as oils, herbs, and supplements, through testing and certification processes.

Ayurveda and Artificial Intelligence: AI can assist in tailoring Ayurvedic treatment plans to individual patient needs by analyzing health data and historical treatment outcomes.

In summary, technology has modernized and complemented Ayurveda in various ways, making it more effective, accessible, and compatible with contemporary healthcare practices.

*****

Case Studies of Various Successful Ayurveda Ventures

Case Study: Patanjali Ayurved Limited

Background: Patanjali Ayurved Limited is a well-known Indian Ayurvedic company founded by Baba Ramdev and Acharya Balkrishna in 2006. The company's mission is to promote the use of Ayurveda, yoga, and traditional Indian medicines for the well-being of individuals.

KEY FACTORS FOR SUCCESS

Authentic Ayurvedic Formulations: Patanjali focuses on producing authentic Ayurvedic products that are based on traditional Ayurvedic principles. Their emphasis on natural ingredients and traditional practices resonated with consumers seeking holistic health solutions.

Strong Leadership and Vision: Baba Ramdev and Acharya Balkrishna, with their deep knowledge of Ayurveda and yoga, provided strong leadership and a clear vision for the company. Their personal branding and endorsements added credibility to the products.

Product Diversification: Patanjali diversified its product range to include a wide variety of consumer goods, including health supplements, personal care products, food items, and more. This diversification appealed to a broader customer base.

Affordable Pricing: The Company offered high-quality Ayurvedic products at competitive prices, making them accessible to a wide range of consumers. This affordability was a key factor in the company's rapid growth.

Aggressive Marketing and Distribution: Patanjali invested heavily in marketing and distribution, making its products widely available in both urban and rural areas. They used a combination of television advertisements and social media to reach consumers.

Transparency and Quality Control: Patanjali maintained transparency in its product manufacturing and quality control processes. This transparency helped build trust with consumers.

Results: Patanjali Ayurved Limited experienced remarkable success and growth. By 2017, it became one of the fastest-growing FMCG (Fast-Moving Consumer Goods) companies in India. Its revenue and market share grew significantly, challenging established multinational brands. The company's success showcased the market potential for Ayurvedic and natural products.

This case study demonstrates how a strong focus on authenticity, leadership, product diversification, pricing, marketing, and quality control can lead to the success of an Ayurveda venture, even in a highly competitive consumer goods industry.

CASE STUDY: SRI SRI TATTVA

Background: Sri Sri Tattva is an Ayurvedic and wellness company founded by spiritual leader Sri Sri Ravi Shankar. The company was established with the goal of promoting holistic wellness through traditional Ayurvedic principles and natural products.

KEY FACTORS FOR SUCCESS

Spiritual Leadership: Sri Sri Ravi Shankar's spiritual influence and reputation lent credibility and trust to the brand. His endorsement and guidance played a significant role in the company's success.

Quality and Authenticity: Sri Sri Tattva prioritizes the quality and authenticity of its Ayurvedic products. They source herbs and ingredients from their own farms and trusted sources to ensure purity and efficacy.

Diverse Product Range: The Company offers a wide range of products, including herbal supplements, personal care items, and food products, catering to various wellness needs of consumers.

Global Expansion: Sri Sri Tattva expanded its presence internationally, making Ayurvedic products accessible to a global market. They established partnerships and retail networks in different countries.

Ayurvedic Consultations: The Company offers Ayurvedic consultation services, allowing customers to receive personalized wellness guidance and product recommendations based on their individual needs.

Social Responsibility: Sri Sri Tattva is involved in various social and environmental initiatives. This commitment to responsible business practices resonates with socially conscious consumers.

Results: Sri Sri Tattva has achieved significant success in the Ayurvedic and wellness industry. The company's emphasis on quality, authenticity, diverse product offerings, global expansion, and a holistic approach to well-being has garnered a loyal customer base both in India and abroad. It has also made Ayurveda more accessible to a global audience.

This case study illustrates how a combination of spiritual leadership, quality, diverse product offerings, international expansion, and a commitment to holistic wellness can lead to the success of an Ayurveda venture. Sri Sri Tattva's integration of Ayurveda into modern wellness practices has contributed to its growth and recognition.

CASE STUDY: BAIDYANATH GROUP

Background: The Baidyanath Group is one of India's oldest and most respected Ayurvedic companies, with a history dating back to 1917. The company was founded by Pandit Ram Dayal Joshi and is known for its traditional Ayurvedic formulations.

KEY FACTORS FOR SUCCESS

Heritage and Legacy: The Baidyanath Group's long-standing legacy and commitment to Ayurveda have earned it a reputation for authenticity and trustworthiness in the Ayurvedic market.

Formulation Expertise: The Company has preserved and continued to develop traditional Ayurvedic formulations, which are based on centuries-old knowledge and practices. This expertise is reflected in their product range.

Modernization and Quality Standards: While maintaining traditional practices, Baidyanath has modernized its manufacturing and quality control processes, ensuring that its products meet contemporary standards.

Research and Development: The Company invests in Ayurvedic research and product development to adapt to evolving consumer needs while remaining true to the principles of Ayurveda.

Extensive Distribution Network: Baidyanath has a well-established distribution network, allowing its products to reach a broad customer base across India and globally.

Ayurvedic Healthcare Centers: The Company operates Ayurvedic healthcare centers and clinics, providing access to expert consultations and Ayurvedic treatments.

Results: The Baidyanath Group has successfully maintained its position as a leading Ayurvedic company for over a century. Its commitment to heritage, formulation expertise, quality, research, distribution, and healthcare services has contributed to its enduring success. The company continues to play a significant role in promoting Ayurveda as a holistic wellness solution.

This case study showcases how the preservation of traditional knowledge, modernization, and a commitment to quality and research can lead to the long-term success of an Ayurveda venture, even in a competitive and evolving market.

CASE STUDY: DABUR INDIA LIMITED

Background: Dabur India Limited is one of the largest and most established Ayurvedic and natural healthcare companies in India. Founded in 1884, Dabur has a rich history of offering Ayurvedic products for various health and wellness needs.

KEY FACTORS FOR SUCCESS

Brand Recognition: Dabur is a well-recognized and trusted brand with a history dating back over a century. The company's long-standing presence has contributed to its strong brand reputation.

Product Diversification: Dabur offers a diverse range of Ayurvedic and natural products, including herbal supplements, personal care items, and foods. This diversification caters to a wide customer base.

Research and Development: The Company invests in Ayurvedic research and modern product development, creating innovative and effective solutions that blend traditional wisdom with contemporary needs.

International Presence: Dabur has successfully expanded its footprint beyond India, making its Ayurvedic products available in various countries, which has contributed to its global success.

Marketing and Promotion: The Company's marketing strategies, including endorsements by celebrities and brand ambassadors, have played a role in creating awareness and interest in its products.

Sustainability Initiatives: Dabur is known for its efforts in promoting sustainable and responsible business practices, which resonate with environmentally conscious consumers.

Results: Dabur India Limited has become a market leader in the Ayurveda and natural healthcare industry. The company's brand recognition, product diversification, research and development, international presence, marketing, and sustainability initiatives have contributed to its success. Dabur's commitment to delivering effective Ayurvedic solutions in a modern context has earned it a strong customer base both in India and internationally.

This case study highlights how a combination of brand legacy, product diversification, research, global expansion, marketing, and sustainability can lead to the sustained success of an Ayurveda venture in the modern world.

CASE STUDY: FOREST ESSENTIALS

Background: Forest Essentials is a luxury Ayurvedic beauty and skincare brand in India, known for its high-quality, natural, and Ayurvedic products. Founded in 2000 by Mira Kulkarni, the company's mission is to revive traditional Ayurvedic beauty rituals and ingredients.

Key Factors For Success

Premium Positioning: Forest Essentials positioned itself as a premium Ayurvedic brand, offering luxury skincare and beauty products that cater to discerning customers seeking natural and effective solutions.

Authentic Formulations: The company places a strong emphasis on authentic Ayurvedic formulations and sources rare, potent herbs and ingredients for its products.

Luxury Packaging: Forest Essentials invests in elegant and eco-friendly packaging, enhancing the overall customer experience and reflecting the brand's premium positioning.

Spa and Retail Presence: The company established its signature stores in India, providing customers with a personalized and immersive shopping experience. It also offers spa treatments that incorporate Ayurvedic principles.

Ethical Sourcing: Forest Essentials is committed to ethical sourcing practices and supports local communities by sourcing ingredients from them.

International Expansion: While primarily an Indian brand, Forest Essentials has made inroads into international markets, catering to a global audience interested in Ayurvedic skincare.

Results: Forest Essentials has achieved remarkable success as a luxury Ayurvedic brand. Its premium positioning, authentic formulations, luxury packaging, retail presence, ethical sourcing, and international expansion have attracted a niche customer base who appreciate the blend of traditional Ayurveda with modern luxury. The company has become a well-recognized name in the beauty and skincare industry.

This case study demonstrates how a focus on premium positioning, authenticity, retail experience, ethical practices, and international reach can lead to the success of an Ayurveda venture in the luxury beauty and skincare sector. Forest Essentials' commitment to Ayurveda and luxury has resonated with consumers seeking both efficacy and indulgence.

CASE STUDY: KAMA AYURVEDA

Background: Kama Ayurveda is an Indian Ayurvedic beauty and wellness brand founded in 2002 by Vivek Sahni, Rajshri Trivedi, and Dave Chang. The brand is known for its natural and authentic Ayurvedic products, emphasizing purity and efficacy.

Key Factors For Success

Ayurvedic Formulations: Kama Ayurveda focuses on authentic Ayurvedic formulations, using natural ingredients and herbs sourced from across India.

Minimalistic Branding: The brand's minimalistic and aesthetic packaging and design appeal to modern consumers who appreciate a blend of traditional wisdom and contemporary presentation.

High-Quality Ingredients: Kama Ayurveda prides itself on sourcing high-quality, organic, and sustainably harvested ingredients, which resonate with environmentally conscious consumers.

Niche Positioning: The brand positions itself as a premium and niche player, catering to a specific segment of consumers looking for natural, chemical-free products.

Online and Offline Presence: Kama Ayurveda has both an online and offline presence, including its own stores and partnerships with luxury retailers, making its products widely available.

Transparency and Certification: The brand maintains transparency about its ingredient sourcing and Ayurvedic processes and has received certifications for its quality standards.

Results: Kama Ayurveda has achieved success as a niche Ayurvedic beauty brand. Its emphasis on authentic Ayurvedic formulations, minimalistic branding, high-quality ingredients, niche positioning, omnichannel presence, and transparency has resonated with modern consumers looking for natural and sustainable alternatives in the beauty and wellness industry.

This case study demonstrates how a focus on authenticity, minimalistic branding, quality ingredients, niche positioning, omni-channel presence, and transparency can lead to the success of an Ayurveda venture in the modern beauty and wellness sector. Kama Ayurveda's blend of tradition and modernity has made it a recognized name in the Ayurvedic beauty industry.

CASE STUDY: VEDIX

Background: Vedix is a personalized Ayurvedic hair and skincare brand founded in India. It was established in 2017 by Chaitanya Nallan and Archit Malik with the goal of offering customized Ayurvedic solutions for individual hair and skin concerns.

Key Factors For Success

Personalization: Vedix stands out by offering personalized Ayurvedic products tailored to each customer's unique hair and skin type. Customers complete an assessment to receive customized formulations.

Data-Driven Approach: The Company employs a data-driven approach to analyze customer responses, Ayurvedic principles, and modern science to create effective personalized formulations.

Online Accessibility: Vedix primarily operates through an e-commerce platform, making it convenient for customers to access their personalized Ayurvedic products.

Ingredient Transparency: Vedix provides detailed information about the ingredients used in their products, enhancing customer trust in the brand.

Ayurvedic Expertise: The Company employs Ayurvedic experts who oversee the formulation and production processes, ensuring the authenticity of the products.

Strong Customer Support: Vedix offers excellent customer support and follow-ups to address any concerns or queries, enhancing the overall customer experience.

Results: Vedix has experienced significant success by merging Ayurvedic principles with modern personalization and e-commerce. Its focus on customization, data-driven approaches, online accessibility, ingredient transparency, Ayurvedic expertise, and customer support has resonated with consumers looking for tailored solutions in their hair and skincare routines.

This case study illustrates how innovation, personalization, technology, and an emphasis on customer needs can lead to the success of an Ayurveda venture, even in a competitive and modern market. Vedix has created a niche for itself by offering truly personalized Ayurvedic solutions for hair and skincare.

CASE STUDY: BIOTIQUE

Background: Biotique is an Indian Ayurvedic beauty and wellness brand founded by Vinita Jain in 1992. The company is known for its wide range of Ayurvedic products that encompass skincare, hair care, and wellness categories.

Key Factors For Success

Traditional Ayurvedic Formulations: Biotique adheres to traditional Ayurvedic principles and utilizes authentic Ayurvedic formulations that include natural ingredients and herbs.

Scientific Validation: While rooted in Ayurveda, Biotique incorporates modern scientific research to validate the effectiveness of its products.

Wide Product Range: The brand offers an extensive range of products, catering to various skincare and haircare needs, as well as wellness products, making it accessible to a broad customer base.

Eco-Friendly Packaging: Biotique focuses on eco-friendly packaging, which resonates with environmentally conscious consumers.

Affordable Pricing: The Company maintains competitive pricing, making Ayurvedic products affordable for a wide demographic.

International Presence: Biotique has expanded its reach internationally, exporting its Ayurvedic products to numerous countries.

Results: Biotique has achieved success as a prominent Ayurvedic brand in the beauty and wellness industry. Its commitment to traditional Ayurvedic formulations, scientific validation, wide product range, eco-friendly packaging, affordability, and international presence has earned it a substantial customer base in India and abroad.

This case study showcases how a blend of traditional wisdom, modern science, sustainability, affordability, and international expansion can lead to the success of an Ayurveda venture. Biotique has successfully combined the rich heritage of Ayurveda with contemporary consumer preferences to become a well-recognized brand in the beauty and wellness market.

CASE STUDY: JIVA AYURVEDA

Background: Jiva Ayurveda is a prominent Ayurvedic healthcare and wellness company founded by Dr. Partap Chauhan in 1992. The company focuses on providing personalized Ayurvedic treatments and products for various health conditions.

Key Factors For Success

Personalized Consultations: Jiva Ayurveda offers personalized online and in-person consultations with Ayurvedic doctors. This one-on-one approach helps tailor treatment plans to individual health needs.

Traditional Ayurvedic Treatments: The Company follows traditional Ayurvedic principles and treatments, incorporating herbal remedies and lifestyle recommendations.

Telemedicine: Jiva Ayurveda embraced telemedicine early on, allowing patients from across the world to access Ayurvedic healthcare services remotely.

Ayurvedic Education: The Company provides Ayurvedic education and training, contributing to the propagation of Ayurvedic knowledge and expertise.

Research and Development: Jiva Ayurveda invests in research and development, aiming to bridge the gap between traditional Ayurveda and modern healthcare.

Quality Control: The Company maintains high standards of quality control in its manufacturing processes, ensuring the authenticity and efficacy of its products.

Results: Jiva Ayurveda has carved a niche in the Ayurvedic healthcare and wellness sector. Its focus on personalized consultations, traditional Ayurvedic treatments, telemedicine, education, research, and quality control has established it as a reliable and respected provider of Ayurvedic healthcare services and products.

This case study illustrates how a commitment to personalized care, modern telemedicine, education, research, and quality standards can lead to the success of an Ayurveda venture. Jiva Ayurveda has contributed to the accessibility and credibility of Ayurveda in the healthcare industry by combining tradition with modern healthcare practices.

CASE STUDY: MAHARISHI AYURVEDA

Background: Maharishi Ayurveda is a globally recognized Ayurvedic company founded by Maharishi Mahesh Yogi in the 1980s. The company's mission is to promote Ayurveda's holistic approach to health and well-being.

Key Factors For Success

Spiritual Guidance: Maharishi Mahesh Yogi's spiritual teachings and his association with transcendental meditation added a unique dimension to the brand and attracted a dedicated following.

Global Reach: Maharishi Ayurveda successfully expanded its presence worldwide, making Ayurvedic products and practices accessible to a global audience.

Ayurvedic Wellness Centers: The Company established Ayurvedic wellness centers that offer consultations, treatments, and holistic programs, providing a comprehensive Ayurvedic experience.

Purity and Authenticity: Maharishi Ayurveda places a strong emphasis on purity and authenticity in its products, sourcing herbs and ingredients from their own organic farms.

Ayurvedic Education: The Company offers Ayurvedic education, including courses and certifications, contributing to the spread of Ayurvedic knowledge.

Sustainability: Maharishi Ayurveda has also embraced sustainable and eco-friendly practices in its operations, aligning with environmentally conscious consumers.

Results: Maharishi Ayurveda has achieved global recognition for its commitment to Ayurvedic principles, its unique spiritual dimension, wellness centers, authenticity, education, and sustainability. The brand has played a significant role in bringing Ayurveda to a worldwide audience.

This case study demonstrates how a blend of spiritual guidance, global reach, holistic wellness centers, purity, education, and sustainability can lead to the success of an Ayurveda venture on an international scale. Maharishi Ayurveda's fusion of traditional Ayurveda with spiritual and global elements has been instrumental in making Ayurveda a global wellness phenomenon.

CASE STUDY: HIMALAYA WELLNESS

Background: Himalaya Wellness, founded in 1930 by M. Manal, is an Indian multinational company that specializes in Ayurvedic healthcare and wellness products. The company is known for its extensive range of herbal and Ayurvedic products for health and personal care.

Key Factors For Success

Traditional Ayurvedic Formulations: Himalaya Wellness maintains a commitment to traditional Ayurvedic formulations, ensuring that its products are based on ancient Ayurvedic knowledge.

Scientific Research: The Company combines traditional wisdom with modern scientific research to validate the effectiveness and safety of its products.

Product Innovation: Himalaya Wellness continuously innovates and expands its product range to cater to various health and wellness needs, including pharmaceuticals, personal care, and wellness supplements.

Quality Control: The Company places a strong emphasis on quality control, utilizing advanced manufacturing processes and adhering to strict quality standards.

Global Expansion: Himalaya Wellness has a significant international presence, exporting its Ayurvedic products to over 90 countries, making it a global Ayurveda brand.

Social Responsibility: The Company engages in various social and environmental initiatives, including sustainable farming practices and community development.

Results: Himalaya Wellness has achieved significant success in the Ayurvedic and wellness industry. Its blend of traditional Ayurvedic knowledge, scientific research, product innovation, quality control, global expansion, and social responsibility has established it as a trusted and globally recognized brand.

This case study illustrates how a combination of traditional wisdom, scientific validation, product diversity, quality standards, global presence, and social responsibility can lead to the success of an Ayurveda venture. Himalaya Wellness has demonstrated how a company can preserve and promote Ayurvedic principles while adapting to the modern needs of consumers on a global scale.

CASE STUDY: KOTTAKKAL ARYA VAIDYA SALA

Background: Kottakkal Arya Vaidya Sala (AVS) is a renowned Ayurvedic institution and healthcare center located in Kottakkal, Kerala, India. Founded in 1902 by the visionary physician P.S. Varier, AVS is dedicated to the practice, research, and propagation of Ayurveda.

Key Factors For Success

Traditional Knowledge Preservation: Kottakkal Arya Vaidya Sala has been instrumental in preserving and propagating traditional Ayurvedic knowledge and practices, including the Ashtavaidya tradition.

Quality Ayurvedic Formulations: The institution produces a wide range of Ayurvedic medicines, known for their high quality and adherence to traditional formulations.

Ayurvedic Hospitals: Kottakkal AVS operates Ayurvedic hospitals, clinics, and research centers, providing authentic Ayurvedic healthcare services.

Educational Initiatives: The institution offers Ayurvedic education through the Kottakkal Ayurveda College and research through its research wing.

International Reach: Kottakkal AVS has expanded its reach to various countries, exporting Ayurvedic products and knowledge.

Sustainability and Organic Farming: The institution practices sustainable and organic farming to source herbs and ingredients for its products, aligning with environmental and health-conscious consumers.

Results: Kottakkal Arya Vaidya Sala has earned global recognition for its dedication to preserving and promoting traditional Ayurvedic knowledge, quality Ayurvedic formulations, healthcare services, education, international reach, and sustainability efforts. It has played a pivotal role in making authentic Ayurveda accessible to people worldwide.

This case study demonstrates how a focus on tradition, quality, healthcare, education, global outreach, and sustainable practices can lead to the success of an Ayurvedic institution. Kottakkal Arya Vaidya Sala's unwavering commitment to the core principles of Ayurveda and its multi-faceted approach have contributed to its enduring success in the field of traditional medicine and healthcare.

CASE STUDY: HAMDARD LABORATORIES (WAKF) LTD.

Background: Hamdard Laboratories is a well-established Indian Unani and Ayurvedic pharmaceutical company with a history dating back to 1906. It was founded by Hakeem Hafiz Abdul

Majeed and is known for its range of herbal and natural health products.

Key Factors For Success

Unani and Ayurvedic Heritage: Hamdard Laboratories is deeply rooted in the Unani and Ayurvedic traditions and is dedicated to preserving and promoting these systems of medicine.

Scientific Research: The Company combines traditional knowledge with scientific research to validate the efficacy and safety of its products.

Diverse Product Range: Hamdard offers a wide range of products, including herbal medicines, wellness supplements, personal care items, and food products, catering to various healthcare and wellness needs.

Strong Distribution Network: The Company has a well-established distribution network, making its products widely available across India and internationally.

Social Initiatives: Hamdard Laboratories is involved in various social and educational initiatives, including the establishment of educational institutions and hospitals.

Quality Assurance: The Company maintains high standards of quality assurance in manufacturing processes to ensure the authenticity and effectiveness of its products.

Results: Hamdard Laboratories has earned a strong reputation as a reliable and authentic provider of Unani and Ayurvedic healthcare products. Its focus on tradition, scientific research, product diversification, distribution, social initiatives, and quality assurance has contributed to its success and recognition.

This case study demonstrates how a commitment to heritage, research, product diversity, distribution, social responsibility, and quality standards can lead to the success of an Ayurveda and Unani venture with a century-long history. Hamdard Laboratories continues to play a significant role in promoting natural and traditional healthcare solutions.

CASE STUDY: VHCA HAIR CLINIC

VHCA HAIR CLINIC: World's 1st Ayurveda Hair Clinic Chain

In the realm of personal aesthetics and self-confidence, hair plays a pivotal role. It's not just a part of our physical appearance, but a reflection of our identity and personality. Recognizing the significance of hair in people's lives, VHCA Hair Clinic has emerged as a beacon of hope and trust, offering comprehensive solutions for various hair-related concerns leveraging the AYURVEDA methodology. With a commitment to excellence, founded in 1998 by renowned Ayurveda Trichologist Dr Mukesh Aggarwal, on the principles of professionalism, innovation, and customer-centricity, VHCA Hair Clinic is backed by research based Ayurveda medicines and cutting-edge technology. From hair loss/thinning/premature greying/dandruff/baldness problems to more complex issues like alopecia areata/trichotillomania and scalp disorders, VHCA Hair Clinic offers a diverse range of treatments tailored to individual needs.

One of the cornerstones of VHCA Hair Clinic's success is its team of experienced and skilled professionals. The clinic boasts a roster of Ayurveda Trichologists & Hair Technicians who possess a deep understanding of the science behind hair health.

VHCA Hair Clinic is known for its state-of-the-art procedures like PRP/GFC/HRP/Laser/Hair Patch/Wig. Furthermore, VHCA Hair Clinic's dedication to transparency and ethical practices has earned it a loyal clientele and has a 95% patient satisfaction.

Challenges

Hair Problems: Many clients suffered from various hair issues, including hair loss, dandruff, premature graying, and scalp conditions.

Competition: The clinic faced competition from conventional hair treatment centers and modern hair transplant clinics.

Awareness: Limited awareness about Ayurvedic treatments for hair care.

Solutions:

Holistic Approach: Dr. Aggarwal and his team employed a holistic approach to diagnose and treat hair problems. They focused on understanding the root causes of hair issues, including diet, lifestyle, and stress.

Customized Treatments: Tailored Ayurvedic treatments were offered to each client based on their unique hair and body constitution (Prakriti).

Herbal Products: The clinic developed its line of Ayurvedic hair care products, including oils, shampoos, and herbal supplements.

Educational Workshops: Regular workshops and seminars were conducted to raise awareness about Ayurvedic practices for hair care.

Online Presence: The clinic maintained an active online presence, offering virtual consultations and informative content on their website and social media.

Results:

Patient Satisfaction: Over the years, the clinic saw a significant increase in patient satisfaction as clients experienced visible improvements in their hair health.

Word of Mouth: Satisfied clients became advocates and referred more individuals to the clinic.

Revenue Growth: The clinic's revenue steadily increased, driven by the sale of their herbal products and services.

Strong Reputation: Dr. Aggarwal's expertise and the clinic's holistic approach contributed to a strong reputation in the community.

Future Directions:

Expansion: The clinic is expending through franchising and has a vision of 100 clinics till 2025 to serve a broader client base.

Research: Dr. Aggarwal and his dedicated research team are doing continue research in ayurvedic trichology.

Digital Outreach: Continue leveraging online platforms for educational content and consultations.

This case study highlights how an Ayurvedic hair clinic successfully addressed hair-related issues through a holistic approach, customized treatments, and a combination of traditional and modern strategies. In conclusion, VHCA Hair Clinic has become synonymous with quality, trust, and expertise in the realm of hair care and restoration.

Resources and References

PROMINENT AYURVEDIC TEXTS:

Charaka Samhita: Authored by Charaka, it is one of the foundational texts of Ayurveda, focusing on general medicine and diagnosis.

Sushruta Samhita: Attributed to Sushruta, this text primarily deals with surgery, including techniques and instruments.

Ashtanga Hridaya: Written by Vagbhata, it's a concise compilation of Ayurvedic knowledge, combining Charaka and Sushruta Samhitas.

Madhava Nidanam: Focusing on diagnostics, this text is authored by Madhavakara.

Bhaishajya Ratnavali: A comprehensive work on Ayurvedic therapeutics authored by Govind Das.

Kashyapa Samhita: Attributed to Kashyapa, it emphasizes pediatrics and gynecology.

Harita Samhita: This text covers toxicology and antidotes.

Yoga Ratnakara: An Ayurvedic text that incorporates knowledge of Ayurveda and yoga practices.

Chakradatta: An ancient text that elaborates on various diseases and their treatments.

Bhavaprakasha: A comprehensive text on Ayurvedic materia medica, authored by Bhavamishra.

Sharngadhara Samhita: Another important text on Ayurvedic pharmacology, which complements the knowledge from Charaka and Sushruta Samhitas.

Nighantu Sangraha: A classic Ayurvedic text that deals with Ayurvedic pharmacology and medicinal plants.

Rasa Ratna Samuchaya: Focuses on Ayurvedic alchemy and the use of minerals and metals in medicine.

Hatha Yoga Pradipika: While not an Ayurvedic text, it contains valuable information on yogic practices and their connection to Ayurveda.

Rasendra Sara Sangraha: An important text on Rasashastra (the science of mercury and metals) and its applications in Ayurvedic medicine.

Sahasrayogam: A compendium of Ayurvedic formulations and prescriptions.

Rasa Tarangini: A classical text on Rasashastra, which deals with the preparation of metallic and mineral medicines.

Shalihotra Samhita: A text dedicated to veterinary medicine and animal care.

Agnivesha Samhita: Often considered one of the oldest texts on Ayurvedic medicine, it's the basis for the Charaka Samhita.

BOOKS BY AYUSH DEPARTMENT

The Ayush Department, part of the Indian government, has published and recommended various books and documents related to traditional Indian systems of medicine and healthcare. Some of these include:

AYURVEDIC PHARMACOPOEIA OF INDIA

NATIONAL AYURVEDIC FORMULARY OF INDIA

Publications on traditional Indian systems of medicine research, education, and practice.

The Ayush Department periodically releases and updates these documents and publications to promote and standardize the practices and medicines of Ayurveda, Yoga, Naturopathy, Unani, Siddha, and Homeopathy in India. You can find these publications on their official website or through authorized bookstores and publications.

National Ayush Morbidity and Standardized Terminologies

Standard Treatment Guidelines for Ayurveda, Siddha, and Unani

GOVERNMENT AYURVEDA ORGANISATIONS

Here are some Indian government Ayurveda organizations:

Ministry of Ayurveda, Yoga & Naturopathy, Unani, Siddha, and Homoeopathy (AYUSH)

Address: MINISTRY OF AYUSH, AYUSH BHAWAN, B Block, GPO Complex, INA, NEW DELHI - 110023

Phone No: 011-24648354

Email: support-moayush@nic.in

Central Council for Research in Ayurvedic Sciences (CCRAS)

Jawahar Lal Nehru Bhartiya Chikitsa Avum Homeopathy Anusandhan Bhavan

No. 61-65, Institutional Area, Opp. 'D' Block, Janakpuri,

New Delhi - 110058 (India)

Telephone: 91-011-28525862/28525897/28525852

National Commission for Indian System of Medicine (NCISM)

Address: 61-65, Institutional Area, Janakpuri "D" Block, New Delhi-110058

Email: secretary@ncismindia.org

Phone: + 91-11-28525464 / +91-11-28522519

National Institute of Ayurveda (NIA)

Jorawar Singh Gate, Amer Road

JAIPUR - 302002 (RAJ.) INDIA

Telephone: 91-141-2635816

All India Institute of Ayurveda (AIIA)

Mathura Road, Goutampuri

Sarita Vihar, Delhi 1100076

Ph: 011-26950401/402

Email: contact-us@aiia.gov.in

National Medicinal Plants Board (NMPB)

Ministry of AYUSH

Government of India

Indian Red Cross Society (IRCS),

Annexe Building, 1st & 2nd floor, 1 Red Cross Road, New Delhi-110001,

Website: www.nmpb.nic.in

Tel: 011-23721840

E-Mail ID: info-nmpb@nic.in

State Ayurvedic Colleges and Hospitals

State Ayurveda Councils and Boards

These organizations play vital roles in promoting traditional Indian systems of medicine, research, education, and healthcare.

INDIAN AYURVEDIC ASSOCIATIONS

There are several Ayurvedic associations in India. Here are a few prominent ones:

All India Ayurvedic Congress (AIAC): AIAC is one of the oldest and most influential Ayurvedic associations in India. It promotes Ayurveda and traditional Indian medicine.

The National Integrated Medical Association (NIMA): is an Indian non-governmental organization of general practitioners educated in Ayurveda system of medicine which includes study of Modern Medicine and knowledge of ayurveda/unani/siddha with scientific approach. NIMA is officially established in 1971 with the motive to promote scientific integration of Modern Medicine & Ancient Indian Medicine i.e. ayurveda/unani/siddha.

National Ayurveda Students and Youth Association (NASYA): NASYA is a youth-oriented organization in India that focuses on promoting Ayurveda among students and young practitioners.

National Ayurvedic Medical Association (NAMA): NAMA is an organization that represents Ayurvedic professionals in India, aiming to advance the practice of Ayurveda.

Ayurveda Medical Association of India (AMAI): AMAI is an association that brings together Ayurvedic doctors and practitioners to promote Ayurvedic healthcare.

International Association for Ayurveda (IAA): While not limited to India, IAA has a presence in the country and promotes Ayurveda worldwide.

Ayurvedic Drug Manufacturers Association (ADMA): ADMA represents the interests of Ayurvedic pharmaceutical companies in India.

Ayurvedic Point of Care (APOC): APOC is a non-profit organization that focuses on Ayurvedic healthcare and research.

Association of Ayurvedic Physicians of Kerala (AAPK): AAPK is a regional association of Ayurvedic doctors in Kerala, a state known for its strong Ayurvedic tradition.

Ayurveda Pharmacy Manufacturers' Association (APMA): APMA represents the interests of Ayurvedic pharmacy manufacturers in the country.

Indian Academy of Ayurveda (IAA): IAA is dedicated to the promotion of Ayurveda through research, education, and advocacy.

Ayurvedic Graduates Medical Association (AGMA): AGMA is an association of Ayurvedic graduates who work to advance the profession and education of Ayurvedic medicine.

All India Association of Ayurvedic Graduates (AIAAG): AIAAG works to protect the rights and interests of Ayurvedic graduates and practitioners.

Indian Institute of Ayurvedic Pharmaceutical Sciences (IIAPS): IIAPS specializes in Ayurvedic pharmaceutical education and research.

Ayurveda Medical Association of India (AMAI): AMAI is another regional association representing Ayurvedic doctors and practitioners in different parts of the country.

Indian Institute of Ayurveda and Integrative Medicine (IIAIM): IIAIM is an institute that focuses on research and education in Ayurveda and integrative medicine.

Ayurveda Hospital Management Association (AHMA): AHMA is dedicated to improving the management and administration of Ayurvedic hospitals and healthcare facilities.

Ayurveda Doctors Association of India (ADAI): ADAI represents Ayurvedic doctors and practitioners across the country, advocating for the profession.

National Ayurvedic Pharmacy Association (NAPA): NAPA is an organization focused on Ayurvedic pharmacy and medication standards.

These organizations continue to play vital roles in the development and promotion of Ayurveda in India.

GLOBAL AYURVEDA ASSOCIATIONS

There are several global Ayurveda associations and organizations that promote and support the practice of Ayurveda worldwide. Some of them include:

World Ayurveda Foundation (WAF): A non-profit organization that aims to promote Ayurveda internationally and facilitate research and education in this field.

International Association of Ayurveda (IAA): A global organization that focuses on the standardization and promotion of Ayurvedic education and practice.

Ayurveda International Academy (AIA): An organization that offers Ayurveda education and certification programs to individuals and professionals worldwide.

National Ayurvedic Medical Association (NAMA): While primarily based in the United States, NAMA has members and partnerships worldwide and is dedicated to promoting Ayurveda and ensuring its integrity.

European Ayurveda Association (EUAA): Focused on promoting Ayurveda in Europe, this association connects Ayurvedic practitioners, educators, and enthusiasts across the continent.

Ayurveda Association of Canada (AAC): This organization is dedicated to promoting Ayurveda in Canada, supporting Ayurvedic practitioners, and providing resources for those interested in Ayurveda.

Ayurveda Association of Singapore (AAOS): Focused on promoting Ayurveda in Singapore and the surrounding region, AAOS works to create awareness about Ayurveda and its benefits.

Ayurveda Association of South Africa (AASA): AASA aims to connect Ayurvedic practitioners, educators, and enthusiasts in South Africa and promote the practice of Ayurveda in the country.

Ayurveda Association of New Zealand: This organization works to support Ayurvedic practitioners, educate the public about Ayurveda, and promote the practice in New Zealand.

Ayurveda Association of Australia: Dedicated to promoting Ayurveda in Australia, this association provides information, resources, and networking opportunities for Ayurvedic practitioners and enthusiasts.

Ayurveda Practitioners' Association in the UK (APA-UK): APA-UK supports Ayurvedic practitioners in the United Kingdom and promotes Ayurveda in the region.

Ayurveda Association of Malaysia: This association focuses on Ayurveda's development and recognition in Malaysia, connecting practitioners and enthusiasts.

Ayurveda Practitioners Association of North America (APNA): APNA serves Ayurvedic practitioners and supporters in North America, facilitating networking and education.

Ayurveda Association of Latin America (AALA): AALA is dedicated to promoting Ayurveda in Latin American countries and connecting practitioners in the region.

Ayurveda Association of the Czech Republic: This organization works to establish Ayurveda in the Czech Republic and offers resources and support for practitioners and enthusiasts.

Association of Ayurvedic Professionals of North America (AAPNA): AAPNA promotes Ayurveda in North America and connects professionals and students in the field.

Ayurveda Association of Ghana: This association seeks to raise awareness of Ayurveda in Ghana and promote its practice and education.

Ayurveda Association of the Netherlands: This organization is dedicated to promoting Ayurveda in the Netherlands and connecting practitioners in the country.

Ayurveda Medical Association of India (AMAI): AMAI represents Ayurvedic medical practitioners in India and advocates for the interests of Ayurvedic doctors.

Ayurveda Practitioners' Association of Sri Lanka: This association supports Ayurvedic practitioners in Sri Lanka and works to promote traditional Ayurvedic medicine in the country.

Ayurveda Association of South Korea: Focused on Ayurveda's promotion in South Korea, this association connects Ayurvedic practitioners and enthusiasts in the country.

Please keep in mind that the status and recognition of these associations may vary, and new organizations may emerge over time. It's a good practice to verify the current status and activities of these associations if you're interested in Ayurveda in specific regions.

Index

W

Y

www.ingramcontent.com/pod-product-compliance
Ingram Content Group UK Ltd.
Pitfield, Milton Keynes, MK11 3LW, UK
UKHW062258290726
14090UKWH00017B/774